CONCUSSION
CARE MANUAL

Concussion Care Manual

A Practical Guide

2ND EDITION

David L. Brody, MD, PhD

Professor of Neurology

Uniformed Services University
of the Health Sciences

Bethesda, Maryland, USA

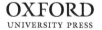

OXFORD
UNIVERSITY PRESS

Oxford University Press is a department of the University of Oxford. It furthers
the University's objective of excellence in research, scholarship, and education
by publishing worldwide. Oxford is a registered trade mark of Oxford University
Press in the UK and certain other countries.

Published in the United States of America by Oxford University Press
198 Madison Avenue, New York, NY 10016, United States of America.

CIP data is on file at the Library of Congress
ISBN 978-0-19-005479-3

9 8 7 6 5 4 3 2 1

Printed by Webcom, Inc., Canada

The opinions and assertions expressed herein are those of Dr. David Brody and do not
necessarily reflect the official policy or position of the Uniformed Services University,
the NIH, or the Department of Defense.

CONTENTS

Acknowledgments from the First Edition

Most importantly, I would like to thank the patients in the concussion clinic at Washington University over the past decade who have been my greatest teachers. I am grateful also to my colleagues Drs. Mick Alexander, Joshua Buck, David Carr, Maurizio Corbetta, David Curfman, Nico Dosenbach, Pouya Fahadan, Mark Halstead, Gerry Gioia, Chris Giza, Esther Hsiao, Nathan Kung, Megumi Vogt, Martin Wice, and Kristy Yuan for helpful suggestions and stimulating discussions. I greatly appreciate the help of Ed Casabar, PharmD and Craig Panner at Oxford University Press for careful editing. Finally, I would like to thank my family for their patience and support during the many Sunday afternoons that I spent working on the manual.

Notes on the Second Edition

Since the first edition was written in 2014, interest around the world in concussion has exploded. Nearly every section of the manual has been updated. There has a been a "quiet revolution" in the field, with a substantial number of randomized controlled trials published in the last 4 years regarding various aspects of concussion care. Still, the patients in concussion clinics in both the military and civilian sectors have remained my greatest teachers, and much of the book is based on what I've learned from them. I am grateful for the additional comments of my colleagues including Louis French, Raquel Gardner, Douglas Katz, Paul McCrory, Daniel Thomas, Michael Xydakis, and Ross Zafonte. I greatly appreciate the editing and technical help of Carly Larkin and Mark Whiting.

PART I

CONCUSSION MANAGEMENT

The Big Picture

Introduction

WHO: This manual is for everyone who treats people with concussion. You don't need to be a brain injury specialist, or a neurologist, or even necessarily a physician to use the manual.

WHY: There are more than 3 million brain injuries each year in the United States and millions more around the world. Most of these injuries are concussions. Most people with concussions get better by themselves quickly within a week or so. We used to think that all of them got better by themselves. Then we thought that less than 10% do not recover quickly by themselves. But now it's clear that 30% or maybe even more can have prolonged symptoms and deficits. Thirty percent is a very large number of people—about 900,000 per year in the United States alone. Much of this manual is written for the people who take care of the 30%. It is also becoming clear that there is not one specific "postconcussion syndrome." Instead, there are many postconcussive paths, and this manual is written to help those who are tasked with figuring this out, one patient at a time. There is also a growing consensus that many of these problems are treatable (Collins et al., Neurosurgery, 2016).

WHAT: This manual is based on my experience and the experiences of my colleagues who, by trial and error, have become experts at identifying, evaluating, and taking care of patients with concussions. This manual is not primarily evidence-based. If it were primarily evidence-based, it would be very short and not very helpful. The evidence base is improving, and this second edition includes multiple updates including recent research findings that were not available when the first edition was written. Nonetheless, there is still a tremendous need for further research and the development of evidence-based guidelines on many topics related to concussion. But this manual is not about research, it is about pragmatic approaches to taking care of patients in the absence of true scientific evidence.

WHERE: This manual is primarily written to be used in an outpatient clinic, but it also can be used on the hospital ward consult service, in the athletic trainer's room, and in a deployed setting. Specific aspects of hospital-based, sports-related, and military concussion treatment are covered.

WHEN: This manual is written to be used "on the fly," right now, without a lot of prior studying or memorization. In that respect, it is modeled after the popular Washington Manual of Diagnostics and Therapeutics that generations of internal medicine house officers have carried in their pockets. Each topic is presented in a clear, succinct manner so that anyone reading the manual can get to the most practical information right away. Some parts of the manual are deliberately redundant for ease of use without a lot of flipping around.

Disclaimer: This manual is meant to supplement, not replace, the knowledge and judgment of medical providers caring for concussion patients. There are no guarantees stated or implied regarding the accuracy or timeliness of any information contained in this manual. Medicine is an evolving art and science, and more up-to-date knowledge may be available elsewhere. With regard to medications, this manual is not intended to be a comprehensive resource, but only meant to outline issues specifically relevant to concussion patients. Specifically, the side effects, dose ranges, indications, and contraindications are not meant to apply to all patients. Only the aspects that are most relevant to concussion patients are presented. Furthermore, this manual should not be interpreted as establishing any sort of medically or legally defined "standard of care."

What Is a Concussion?

A concussion is a traumatic brain injury, but not an immediately life-threatening one. There is no severe brain swelling that requires intensive care-unit management and no bleeding that requires brain surgery. But a concussion is definitely a traumatic injury to the brain. Some use the term "mild" traumatic brain injury to describe concussion, but mild means "soft" or "gentle" like mild soap or a mild-mannered person. There is nothing "mild" about the experience for many patients.

A traumatic brain injury means that there has been a sudden force applied to the brain from outside. Examples include something hitting the head (e.g., another person, a baseball, or a falling rock), the head hitting something (e.g., the ground, a wall, or a car windshield), or the head rotating fast (as in many motor vehicle accidents). But not every force causes a concussion. In fact, most do not. The scalp, skull, and dura do a pretty good job protecting our brains from most of what happens to us on a daily basis. *A traumatic brain injury means that the force applied to the brain caused a disruption in the brain's structure, an impairment of the brain's function, or both.* Examples of disruption of the brain's structure include bleeding, bruising, and swelling, which can be seen on computed tomography (CT) scans and magnetic resonance imaging (MRI) scans. More commonly, however, concussion may involve tearing of axons, which usually cannot be seen on CT scans and MRI scans. *This is important. Just because a CT or MRI scan is negative does not mean that there has not been a concussion. Traumatic brain injury, especially concussion, is a clinical diagnosis, not based on any lab test or scan.* Impairments in brain function caused by force applied to the brain sufficient to cause concussion usually involve loss of consciousness,

TABLE 2.1 Differentiating Concussion from More Severe Traumatic Brain Injury and Other Disorders

	Concussion	Moderate-to-Severe Traumatic Brain Injury	Other Disorders
Loss of consciousness	None or less than 30 minutes	Often more than 30 minutes	May be present, but not directly due to injury (e.g., syncope, seizure)
Amnesia	Up to 24 hours	Often more than 24 hours	May be due to other causes (e.g., toxic substances, delirium, postictal state)
Headache	Often present	Often present, when assessable	Often present (nonspecific)
Glasgow Coma Scale	13–15	9–12 (moderate) or 3–8 (severe)	Variable
CT scan	Normal	Often abnormal with characteristic findings	Usually normal or with abnormalities characteristic of other disorders

amnesia, disorientation, or problems with balance and coordination. Other impairments in brain function can include changes in vision—seeing things in a distorted fashion ("seeing stars")—confusion, inappropriate behavior (running the wrong way on the football field), or changes in emotion. This is where some medical knowledge is required: An injury that causes burning pain in all

TABLE 2.2 The Glasgow Coma Scale

Eye response

4	Opens eyes spontaneously
3	Opens eyes in response to speech
2	Opens eyes in response to painful stimulation
1	Does not open eyes in response to any stimulation

Motor response

6	Follows commands
5	Makes localized movement in response to painful stimulation
4	Makes nonpurposeful movement in response to noxious stimulation
3	Flexes upper extremities and extends lower extremities in response to pain
2	Extends all extremities in response to pain
1	Makes no response to noxious stimuli

Verbal response	*(Cannot assess in an intubated patient)*
5	Oriented to person, place, and time
4	Confused responses
3	Inappropriate words
2	Incomprehensible sounds
1	No verbal response

Adapted from Teasdale et al., Lancet, 1974.

4 limbs and weakness of both legs is probably a "stinger" or cervical spine injury, not a concussion. Likewise, weakness in one arm after a blow to the head and shoulder is more likely a peripheral nerve injury rather than a concussion (see Table 2.1). Headaches are common after concussion, but also common after injuries to the head that do not cause impairment in brain function. So, headache after an injury does not automatically mean that the injury caused

concussion. Ringing in the ears and loss of balance after a blast could be due to inner ear damage rather than concussion.

For many patients with traumatic brain injury, providers will assess the initial severity of injury using the Glasgow Coma Scale (GCS) (Table 2.2). Typically, patients with concussion have GCS scores between 13 and 15. Lower GCS, abnormal findings on CT, unconsciousness more than 30 minutes, or amnesia more than 24 hours typically indicate a more severe form of traumatic brain injury unless there was another cause for the reduced GCS.

3

How Do You Make the Diagnosis of Concussion?

You need a *reliable history* of 2 things:

(1) An acute external physical force applied to the brain

AND

(2) An impairment in the function of the brain directly caused by the external physical force.
  - One or the other is not enough. You need both.
  - You do not need a scan or lab test to make the diagnosis. No scan or test can "rule in" or "rule out" concussion. The blood tests and electroencephalogram (EEG)-based tests recently approved by the U. S. Food and Drug Administration are useful for determining whether a patient needs a computed tomography (CT) scan; they cannot, however, reliably be used to make a diagnosis of concussion (despite reports in the popular press).
  - You do not need to perform a detailed neurological exam to make the diagnosis. The neurological exam is usually unremarkable except for immediately after the concussion. No exam findings can definitively "rule in" or "rule out" concussion.
  - Helmet sensors or other impact sensors cannot be used to make a diagnosis of concussion. The relationship between sensor data and actual concussion is still quite weak. A concussion can occur with modest sensor-recorded forces, and people can have high sensor-recorded forces

without experiencing concussion or any other detectible injury.

(A) *How do you know whether the history is reliable?* This takes judgment and a bit of insight, but it is usually not too hard. Most people who need help tell the truth to their medical providers. If they are not telling the truth, it is usually apparent pretty quickly. A collateral source helps a lot. This means someone else who either witnessed the event, or more commonly saw the person afterward and observed the effects. Often, the patient doesn't remember exactly what happened. Of course not. Amnesia is one of the common features of concussion. *The collateral source is key.* You have not gotten the history until you've gotten a reliable collateral history. The certainty of your diagnosis is directly proportional to the quality of your collateral history. It is OK to say, "possible concussion—pending further collateral source information." You should still treat the patient, but reserve final judgment about the cause of the patient's symptoms until you have gotten a reliable history.

(B) *What are some examples of external physical forces that typically cause concussion?*

  - Motor vehicle crashes that produce damage to the vehicles involved.
  - Falls from more than standing height, such as down a flight of stairs, off a ladder, from a horse, or out of a tree.
  - Falls from standing height or less where the person is not able to catch himself or herself, such as slipping on the ice, falling while drunk, being pushed or thrown violently.
  - Contact sports such as football, rugby, hockey, lacrosse, boxing, and mixed martial arts.
  - Assault, such as being struck in the head with a blunt object, punched, kicked, or head-butted.
  - Direct blast exposure closer than safe standoff distance. Safe distance is a controversial topic, so it's OK to say, "possible concussion versus subconcussive exposure"

after a blast when it's not clear. Then treat the patient's symptoms and deficits.

- A glancing or grazing bullet (penetrating injuries such as gunshot wounds cause more severe traumatic brain injuries).
- Hard shaking in babies and very young children.

(C) *What are some examples of external physical forces that typically DO NOT cause concussion?*

- Bumping the head against something during normal activities.
- Relatively trivial motor vehicle crashes that do not damage the vehicle or set off any of the safety devices (though these can still sometimes cause whiplash injuries to the neck).
- Falls that do not involve directly striking the head.
- Falls from standing height or less where the person is able to catch himself.
- Shaking, unless the shaking is especially violent or also results in impact.
- Heading a soccer ball (though the effects of large numbers of headers in the long term are not yet clear).
- Blast exposure from safe standoff distances (though again the effects of large numbers of subconcussive blast exposures in the long term are not yet clear).

(D) *How do you tell whether the external physical force caused the impairment in brain function?*

Again, judgment and a bit of insight are key. Typically, all of the following are true:

(1) The impairment in brain function occurs immediately after the event. For example, the patient lost consciousness right after falling and hitting her head. Make sure she didn't lose consciousness from something else (such as fainting or a seizure), and then fell and hit her head.

(2) The impairment is worst immediately after the event, then gradually improves. For example, the patient has a gap in memory for 15 minutes after the car crash, remembers bits and pieces of the ambulance ride, and then remembers everything that happened at the hospital. Some symptoms, such as migraine headaches and depression, can appear later, but *at least some impairment in brain function at the time of the injury is required for the diagnosis of concussion.*

(3) There is no other obvious explanation for the impairment. Specifically, the patient did not have the impairment prior to injury, and there wasn't another cause, such as exposure to toxins or an anoxic injury. Sometimes it just isn't clear whether the loss of consciousness was due to head injury or due to something else. Examples of other causes of loss of consciousness include low blood pressure caused by bleeding from other injuries, fainting (syncope), cardiac arrhythmia, low blood sugar, and many others. Amnesia can sometimes be caused by the shock of the event itself, and confusion can happen to anyone in the "'fog of war." Headache can have many causes. Ringing in the ears and loss of balance can be caused by inner ear damage, rather than brain injury.

Again, it is OK to reserve judgment about the cause, call it "possible concussion" or "probable concussion," and start treating the patient's symptoms right away while you gather more information over time.

4

Diagnosis of Sport Concussion

In the setting of a sporting event, it is much more likely that the event itself and its effects on the patient will have been directly witnessed. Get a collateral source history from those who actually observed the event and ask the following questions:

1. Did the patient lose consciousness? If so, for how long?
2. Were there any convulsions (body twitching and jerking) and if so, how long did they last?
3. Did anyone test the patient's memory with questions such as, Who is your team playing? What happened in the last part of the game or practice? What period is this? What happened in your team's previous competition?
4. Did the patient behave in an odd fashion? If so, for how long?
5. Is there any sideline video?
6. Did the patient have any cognitive testing (such as SCAT, ImPACT, HeadMinder) and if so, what were the results? Were they impaired compared to baseline?
7. Was the patient's balance formally tested (e.g., by using the Balance Error Scoring System), and if so, what were the results?
8. Did the patient have Vestibular Ocular Motor Screening (VOMS), and if so, what were the results?

With this information, the diagnosis can often be made much more accurately than when the event was not witnessed.

Again, you do not need a scan or lab test to make the diagnosis.

Again, helmet sensors or other impact sensors cannot be used to make a diagnosis of concussion. The relationship between sensor data and actual concussion is still quite weak. A concussion can occur with modest sensor-recorded forces, and people can undergo high sensor-recorded forces without experiencing concussion or any other detectible injury.

Importantly, all kinds of sporting events can result in concussion. Not just boxing, football, hockey, and rugby, but also soccer, basketball, baseball, softball, equestrian sports, diving, bicycle racing, and many others are associated with increased risk of concussion. However, heading the ball in soccer has NOT been demonstrated to cause concussion. Most soccer concussions come from collisions with another player or a goal post. The long-term effects of heading the ball or other subconcussive head impacts have not been determined with certainty. Recent research in former American college football players indicates that the total number of lifetime subconcussive impacts may be a stronger predictor of late-life neurological and behavioral difficulties than the number of concussions (Montenigro et al., J Neurotrauma, 2017). When in doubt, treat the patient's symptoms and reserve judgment about the cause.

Use the Sport Concussion Assessment Tool 5th Edition (SCAT5) to guide a standard *acute* evaluation and management of sport-related concussion.

https://bjsm.bmj.com/content/bjsports/early/2017/04/26/bjsports-2017-097506SCAT5.full.pdf

This takes 10 to 15 minutes and should be performed after the athlete is rested, ideally when heart rate is back to normal baseline. This version of the assessment tool has multiple word lists, so that it would be very hard for an athlete to memorize them all in advance (Echimedia et al., British Journal of Sports Medicine, 2017). https://bjsm.bmj.com/content/51/11/848

The SCAT5 has appropriate advice for initial management, based on an expert consensus group (McCrory et al., British Journal of Sports Medicine, 2017).

Later, a more individualized approach may be needed.

Consider performing a short screening test such as the VOMS. This test involves asking whether symptoms worsen after testing smooth pursuit eye movements, saccadic eye movements, near point convergence, vestibular ocular reflex, and visual motion sensitivity. The best way to learn to perform VOMS is by watching a video.

http://rethinkconcussions.upmc.com/2016/10/what-is-voms/

The detailed instructions can be found online.

https://www.physiotherapyalberta.ca/files/vomstool.pdf

The VOMS is reportedly 90% accurate in identifying adolescent patients with concussion an average of 5 days after sport-related injury. How accurate it is in other settings isn't well known. Either way, if there is a reliable history or acute external physical force applied to the brain AND impairment in the function of the brain directly caused by the external physical force, it's still most likely a concussion, even if the VOMS is normal.

A note about helmets: Helmets are designed to reduce skull fractures and more severe traumatic brain injuries such as intracerebral hemorrhages and contusions. But helmets do little to reduce the risk of concussion. Concussion is mainly caused by rotational acceleration of the head, which is not prevented by wearing a helmet. In contrast, airbags for bicyclists that deploy from a device worn around the neck probably do substantially reduce rotational acceleration. At present, these airbags for bicyclists are available for sale in Europe but not in the United States.

See Chapter 30 for specific guidance in managing return to contact sports after concussion.

See Chapters 34 to 35 for special topics in adolescents and children.

See Chapter 36 for guidance in managing contact sport athletes and others with multiple concussions.

5

Which Problems Do You Address First?

Concussion patients often have a lot of things going on at the same time. Consider these three principles:

(1) Ask the patient what's bothering him the most. Often it is pain. Migraine headaches, for example, can be terrible. Try to deeply understand the patient's life to figure out what matters most.

(2) Ask the collateral source what's causing the most problems in the patient's life? Often it is mood instability. "He's not the same person" is a common complaint. Sometimes, the most important problems following concussion are not immediately apparent to the patient.

(3) Look for the "top of the cascade": one single problem that is the root cause of one or more additional problems. For example, sleep disruption can in turn worsen memory, attention, pain, mood disorders, and many other symptoms. Major depression can impair virtually every aspect of life, including energy, sleep, pain, attention, and memory.

6

General Treatment Strategies

Top 10 General Priorities

(1) Do one thing at a time. Otherwise you will never figure out what caused what. It is OK to lay out a treatment plan on the first visit, then go through the steps one at a time on subsequent visits or by phone or e-mail.

(2) Educate and comfort. We can cure rarely, and treat sometimes, but we can educate and comfort always. Early education and reassurance can provide substantial benefit in reducing secondary anxiety.

(3) Give an honest prognosis with a positive spin. Avoid the "nocebo" effect that comes from setting an expectation of sickness. Offer a sense of perspective. Most people recover well from concussion. Even those who haven't been recovering quickly on their own can benefit from specific treatments.

(4) Offer rehabilitative therapy and lifestyle modification interventions as well as medications. Medications are only "one-third of the pie." Rehabilitative therapy and lifestyle modifications are the other two-thirds.

(5) Stop or taper impairing medications before adding new ones.

(6) Minimize side effects of medications. Assess for side effects specifically on each visit. A concussed person can be more vulnerable to cognitive impairment, fatigue, or mood destabilization from medications than an uninjured person.

(7) Use a healthy dose of Vitamin P ("placebo") in an appropriate way ("If this is the right medication for you, it is really going to help over the next 4 to 6 weeks. Hang in there!")

(8) Under the right circumstances, it's OK to use a big dose of Vitamin S (the "'therapeutic scare'") also. ("If you don't stop drinking alcohol, these headaches are never going to get better and none of the medicines are going to work the way they are supposed to work.")

(9) Offer follow-up and appropriate referrals. Identify the local experts in each of the specific concerns related to your concussion patients. If you can't send the patient, call or e-mail the expert for "curbside consult" advice.

(10) Support the family. Acknowledge that it is difficult for them. Tell them how important they are for the patient's recovery. Complex concussions can be a big strain on marriages and other relationships. However, patients who get divorced or estranged from family and friends often do substantially worse in the long term.

PART II

HOW TO MANAGE SPECIFIC PROBLEMS

7

Headaches

Headaches are the most common sustained symptom after concussion, and often one of the most disabling symptoms in the subgroup of patients who don't recover quickly (i.e., the ones on whom you will focus most of your attention). See Figure 7.1.

In the first 48 hours after concussion, ibuprofen, acetaminophen, or both are usually recommended. The authors of an open-label, randomized trial involving 8- to 18-year-olds with concussion reported that ibuprofen, acetaminophen, or both improved headaches compared to no treatment. Ibuprofen or the combination of both ibuprofen and acetaminophen increased the likelihood of returning to school within 1 week (Petrelli et al., Pediatrics and Child Health, 2017). Another less commonly used option is hypertonic saline; 10 mL/kg of 3% saline reduced immediate headache and headaches over the first 2 to 3 days compared to normal saline in a pediatric emergency department trial (Lumba-Brown et al., Pediatric Emergency Care, 2014).

A lot of patients, however, go on to have further headaches over the following months to years, and ibuprofen and acetaminophen are often not enough.

First Rule: Triage Is More Important than Diagnosis

How do you tell if the headache is a sign of something dangerous or not?

Most of the time after a brain injury, a headache is not a harbinger of impending demise. Usually you will be focusing on finding the

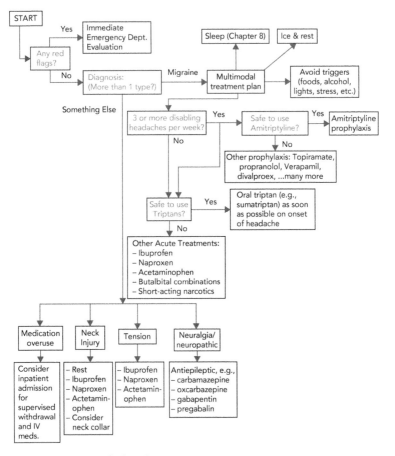

FIGURE 7.1 Headache after concussion.

right combination of medications and lifestyle modifications. But occasionally there is something dangerous going on.

(1) Take a careful history. Don't just listen; this could take all day and not get you anywhere. You have to actively take the history by asking specific hypothesis-testing questions.

   a. "Is it positional?" "Does your headache immediately get much worse when you stand up, and much better when you lie down?" If so, this is a red flag for low cerebrospinal fluid (CSF) pressure headache. This could be caused by a CSF leak, such as from a cribriform plate fracture in the head or thecal sac rupture in the neck or back. The patient needs a lumbar puncture right away with careful measurement of opening pressure. If the pressure is truly low, a careful evaluation for a leak should be performed. This can turn into meningitis if you don't catch it early. It's OK to perform lumbar punctures on a large number of patients to prevent one case of meningitis. Many patients will turn out to have migraine, which also can be positional, but if you get a really strong history, it's better to be safe than sorry.

b. "Is it the other way? Does it get better when you stand up and is it worse when you lie down or worse first thing in the morning?" This is a red flag for the opposite problem: high intracranial pressure. High pressure can be due to mass effect like an expanding subdural or epidural hematoma (sometimes missed on the initial scan), delayed cerebral edema, or hydrocephalus. The patient needs a computed tomography (CT) scan of the head and possibly a lumbar puncture. Again, it is OK to scan a large number of patients to catch one serious case. A lot will turn out to be sleep apnea or musculoskeletal neck problems.

c. "Any unusual fluid leaking from the nose or ears?" This could be a cerebrospinal fluid leak. Again, a CSF leak needs to be addressed right away before it turns into meningitis.

d. "Any loss of vision in one eye?" Even though not directly related to concussion, you never want to miss a case of temporal arteritis. If there is concern, get a blood erythrocyte sedimentation rate (ESR) right away. If it is high, have ophthalmology see the patient right away.

e. "Any weakness, severe numbness, or tingling in the arms and legs, bowel or bladder incontinence?" This could indicate a cervical spine injury, which sometimes presents as head and neck pain. Get cervical spine X-rays, a CT scan of the neck, or a magnetic resonance imaging (MRI) scan of the neck right away.

(2) Examine the patient. This is important. You can't do it over the phone. You need to see the patient in person. You are looking for "red flags" that would indicate that the patient needs to go to the emergency room for a scan and further evaluation. Main points:

a. *Severity.* A really severely distressed patient who is moaning or writhing in pain is more likely to have something bad going on than one who is calm or primarily anxious-looking. For triage, observation of the patient is more important that what the patient says about the subjective severity of the headache.

b. *Mental status.* If mental status is off from baseline and there isn't another good reason for it, send the patient for a CT scan right away. It could be a bleed, edema, postictal state, infection, intoxication, or many other things. You can't tell for sure in a patient whose mental status is altered.

c. *Eye movements.* If the patient can't move her eyes upward (upgaze palsy), this could be a sign of increased intracranial pressure. Some older patients, however, can't do this well at baseline, so hopefully there is a previous exam documented. A few people have congenital problems with upgaze that aren't caused by injury; they usually have jumpy side-to-side eye movements (horizontal nystagmus) when trying to look up. This runs in families and the patient or collateral source is likely to know about it. Ask the patient or the collateral source if the problem was there before the injury. If so, don't worry about it. Likewise, if one eye has trouble moving outward (6th nerve palsy) this can be a sign of increased intracranial pressure. Some people, however, have had childhood strabismus, which can decompensate after traumatic brain injury. A trick: Use a $20 bill or a small mirror to test eye movements. Your finger really isn't that interesting and a lot of concussion patients are inattentive. Bottom line: A change in eye movements from baseline after injury could be a problem, but you've got to know what the baseline was.

d. *Pupils.* A dilated and unreactive pupil can be a sign of herniation *in a comatose or obtunded patient.* If the patient's mental status is normal, it is usually something benign like medication getting into the eye or Adie's tonic pupil (an intermittent condition of no real clinical significance). Rarely an unruptured aneurysm or cranial nerve palsy can cause a dilated pupil, but these can be handled nonurgently. So, mental status comes first.

e. *Walking.* If the patient can't walk normally, and this is a change from baseline, something bad may be going on. Maybe a posterior fossa bleed, maybe cerebral edema. The patient needs a CT scan.

f. *The neck.* It takes just a second, but a stiff neck raises a concern for meningitis. Meningitis can be caused by a cerebrospinal fluid leak after head trauma, for example. Stiff neck can come before fever or change in mental status. If the patient has a stiff neck, get a CT scan and a lumbar puncture right away.

g. DOCUMENT YOUR EXAM. If it is normal, make it clear exactly what you did and what you found, so that the next time something happens, the patient's baseline status will be clear. You don't have to use specialized neurological vocabulary. It's OK to say, "the up-down and side-to-side eye movements were normal."

(3) In ambiguous cases, especially when headaches are worsening over time, consider an evaluation for *cerebral sinus vein thrombosis*. Usually this is done with a magnetic resonance (MR) venogram. Head trauma in the preceding month is the most common risk factor, even in patients without additional hormonal or genetic risk factors. Pregnant and postpartum women, and those with other hypercoagulable states are at especially high risk. Cerebral sinus vein thrombosis can be a cause of refractory headaches and is treatable with anticoagulation. It can lead to stroke if not treated, so don't wait. It's OK to order a lot of MR venograms in patients with worsening headaches to catch a few cases of cerebral sinus thrombosis.

If you have established that there are no red flags, then the patient is not going to be someone else's problem for the moment. At this point you need to make a diagnosis.

Second Rule: Migraines Are Really Common after Concussion; An Atypical Presentation of Migraine Is Still More Likely than Most Other Types of Headaches

For example, moderately intense pain after concussion that affects the whole head and does not throb but is accompanied by nausea is still more likely to be migraine than anything else.

Third Rule: Patients Can Have More than One Type of Headache at the Same Time

Don't stop once you've gotten one diagnosis. A patient can have migraine, tension headache, and trigeminal neuralgia all at the same time.

Fourth Rule: Patients with Medication Overuse Headache Aren't Going to Get Better from Anything You Do until the Medication Overuse Is Addressed

Please see the section on treatment of medication overuse headaches later in this chapter.

Most Common Headache Diagnoses

Migraine

(1) Severity: Most migraines are moderate to severe. Ask how much the headache affects daily life, rather than using the 1 to 10 scale. "Mild" means nonimpairing, "moderate" means impairing but nondisabling, and "severe" means disabling.

(2) Nausea or vomiting: Very typical for migraine but not required for the diagnosis.

(3) Photophobia: "Do bright lights hurt your eyes more than usual when you have one of these headaches?" Sometimes this is obvious—they come into the exam room with sunglasses. One concussion clinic had exam rooms lit with Christmas lights rather than fluorescents because photophobia is so common.

(4) Phonophobia: "Do loud noises bother you more than usual when you have one these headaches?" This may be even worse in postconcussive migraine than in regular migraine.

(5) Osmophobia: "Do smells bother you more than usual with the headache?"

(6) Cogniphobia: "Does it hurt your head to think or concentrate?"

NOTE: Cogniphobia may be more common in concussion-related migraine than in ordinary migraine.

Cogniphobia may be associated with poor or erratic performance on neuropsychological testing, including poor performance on tests of effort (Silverberg, Journal of Neurotrauma, 2017).

(7) Allodynia: "Does it hurt to touch your face, head, or neck?" Hypersensitivity to light touch can be a warning sign that a migraine is coming on, or part of the migraine itself.

(8) Neurological aura (not necessary for diagnosis, but very characteristic) including a wide range of experiences such as seeing bright spots of jagged colored lines, other changes in vision, confusion, balance impairment, vertigo, anxiety, and less commonly focal neurological deficits mimicking a transient ischemic attack.

> NOTE: Some concussion patients may have neurological auras without actual headache. This can pose a diagnostic dilemma but respond to the same treatments as typical migraine headaches. See below.

(9) Exercise-related? This is common after concussion, especially with activity that increases intra-abdominal pressure.

(10) Location? Typically unilateral but can be bilateral or diffuse.

(11) Character? Usually throbbing, but not always. Sometimes it just hurts.

Neuralgia (trigeminal, occipital, etc.), also known as "neuropathic" head pain

(1) A shooting, electrical painful sensation in a specific part of the head or face.

(2) Follows the distribution of a specific cranial nerve or branch on one side. Most common are the trigeminal nerve branches V1 (forehead and top of the head, back to the ear), V2 (cheek and nose, down to the upper jaw).

(3) Usually lasts just a few seconds but can last longer.

(4) Often very intense.

(5) Sometimes can be triggered by light touch or pressure to a particular area of the head or face.

(6) Sometimes, but not always, in a location that makes sense based on the injury. For example, trigeminal neuralgia in the V2 distribution after an orbital floor fracture.

Tension

(1) Typical dull pain.
(2) Often poorly localized.
(3) Accompanied by muscle tension (though virtually all pain is accompanied by some muscle tension).
(4) Often a headache that doesn't have any of the characteristics of the other types.

Medication Overuse

(1) Typically someone who has been taking high doses of pain medications more than 15 days per month for at least 3 months. Common offenders include NSAIDs (e.g., ibuprofen, naproxen), acetaminophen, triptans, butalbital combinations, and narcotics.
(2) Always present, never completely goes away even with medication.
(3) Often quite nonspecific in character.
(4) Usually moderate in severity, on the edge of tolerable with medication.
(5) Headaches get worse when stopping the medication.

Musculoskeletal Neck Injury. The same forces that cause concussion can also injure the neck, in what is commonly called "whiplash."

(1) Neck pain radiating to the back of the head.
(2) Pain on turning or flexing the head.
(3) Tenderness at the junction between the head and neck.
(4) Pain on pressing the head forward or backward isometrically.

(5) There is sometimes subluxation or misalignment on cervical spine X-rays, CT-scans, or MRI, but these imaging findings rarely influence treatment.

Cluster Headache

(1) Intense, brief pain often in a specific part of the face.
(2) Accompanied by one eye watering, nose running, blood vessels in the eyes dilated and red, sometimes flushing (all of these are examples of autonomic hyperactivity).
(3) Come in clusters: several headaches in the same day, week, or month, then a period of relatively few headaches. But migraines can come in clusters, too, often triggered by some kind of stress.

Other headaches, not characteristic of any of the above

Re-evaluate next visit. Ask the patient and family to keep a diary of the headache characteristics and bring it to the next visit. This may help clarify the diagnosis, given that it can be difficult to recall the exact characteristics of the headaches after they have resolved.

Next, the hard part: finding the right treatment. Some of this is trial and error, but the criteria below can be used to make an educated guess about where to start.

For all types of pain, consider a combination of rehabilitative therapies and lifestyle modifications in addition to medications. There is emerging evidence that cognitive behavioral therapy, either in person or by telephone, can reduce pain intensity, and even more importantly, reduce pain interference with activities. Good-quality education about pain can also be effective. These approaches can be especially important for people with chronic pain, pain of many types, and maladaptive "catastrophizing" responses to pain.

Generally, avoid marijuana. Although there are many claims that marijuana improves headaches, in truth very little is known about this. There are also many examples of markedly impaired cognitive function, weight gain, and worsening fatigue due to marijuana. It isn't clear whether these effects are due to impurities or other drugs added to make it more addictive. As marijuana becomes legal and more carefully regulated, more will be learned about its role in concussion management.

Acute Migraine Treatment

(1) Nonpharmacological measures
   a. Optimize sleep (Chapter 8). Migraine headaches rarely respond fully to medication when there is substantial sleep deprivation.
   b. Reduce exposure to the triggers: bright light, loud noise, harsh smells, specific foods, extreme temperatures. Prescribe sunglasses, earplugs, a mask, time off work, etc.
   c. Tell the patient to lie down in a dark, quiet room. A short nap often relieves migraine. A note to the patient's employer or school can help ensure that this will be allowed.
   d. Ice pack to the head or neck for 15 minutes.
   e. Meditation or progressive relaxation exercises. These take practice in advance—the patient will be unlikely to do them for the first time in the middle of a migraine.
   f. Refer the patient to a psychologist or counselor for cognitive behavioral therapy to reduce pain interference with activities.
(2) Triptans
   a. There are a wide range of choices and doses available. Our most common prescription is "Sumatriptan 50 mg po as soon as possible on onset of headache, may repeat after 2 hours. No more than 200 mg per 24 hours. #9." Any of the other oral triptan pills are acceptable, as there are no clear advantages or disadvantages other than cost and what is covered by the patient's insurance.
   b. For slightly faster onset or for patients so nauseated they cannot swallow a pill, consider a rapidly dissolving oral

form such as rizatriptan orally disintegrating tablets (Maxalt MLT), typical dose 10 mg.

c. For substantially faster onset, consider a nasal spray, such as sumatriptan (Imitrex Nasal Spray) 5 or 20 mg per spray. Warn the patient that this can taste terrible.

d. If a triptan alone has an incomplete benefit, consider a combination of a triptan along with high dose over-the-counter pain medication (e.g., 600 mg ibuprofen, 1000 mg acetaminophen). This combination is not contraindicated. Just the opposite; it is often synergistic.

e. Side effects

   i. Coronary and cerebral vasoconstriction causing angina, myocardial infarction, transient ischemic attack, or ischemic stroke. This is extremely rare in patients without coronary artery disease or cerebrovascular disease. Triptans are generally safe in otherwise healthy patients.

   ii. Tightening sensation in the neck or chest that can be alarming but not dangerous. Warn the patient to avoid anxiety.

   iii. Abdominal discomfort or diarrhea uncommonly.

There is extremely low risk of serotonin syndrome when triptans are used along with serotonin specific reuptake inhibitors such as paroxetine and fluoxetine. So even if the pharmacist flags a drug–drug interaction, it's usually OK to go ahead (Chapter 11).

f. Advantages

   i. Very effective

   ii. Not habit forming

   iii. No street value

   iv. No refill hassles

   v. Patients can and should carry these with them at all times to be able to take immediately on onset of headache or aura.

g. Contraindications: coronary artery disease, cerebrovascular disease. *If there are any doubts, image the cerebral vessels (MR angiogram, CT angiogram) and get a cardiac stress test.* Better to sort this out early and get the patient the best treatment right away.

(3) Over-the-counter analgesics and nonsteroidal anti-inflammatory agents (NSAIDS). Generally somewhat less effective compared with triptans, but they are the first-line treatment for patients in whom triptans are contraindicated or too expensive.

  a. Ibuprofen (Motrin and others) 600 mg po as soon as possible on onset of headache.

  b. Acetaminophen (Tylenol and others) 1000 mg po as soon as possible on onset of headache.

  c. Naproxen (Aleve and others) 220 to 550 mg po as soon as possible on onset of headache.

  d. Numerous other possibilities, including combinations of NSAIDs with caffeine (e.g., Excedrin Migraine: acetaminophen + aspirin + caffeine).

  e. Advantages
    i. Inexpensive
    ii. No hassles

  f. Contraindications:
    i. NSAIDS: Renal dysfunction
    ii. History of NSAID-related gastrointestinal (GI) bleeding
    iii. Gastric ulcer disease (though adding anti-acid therapy sometimes helps)
    iv. NSAIDs: Recent long bone fracture or major orthopedic surgery (ask the surgeon)
    v. Acetaminophen (Tylenol) contraindicated in liver failure

(4) Butalbital combinations

  a. Dosing: Fioricet (butalbital 50 mg/acetaminophen 325 mg/caffeine 40 mg) 1 to 2 tabs po q 4 hrs prn severe headache #30 refills 0.

      b. Alternative: many other combinations (Fiorinal with 325 mg aspirin instead of acetaminophen)

      c. Advantages

         i. Very effective for pain

        ii. Some anxiety relieving effects as well

      d. Disadvantages

         i. Substantial risk of medication overuse headache. Limit use to most severe headaches.

        ii. Habit forming in some.

       iii. Tolerance develops in some.

       iv. Some street value—risk of being lost, stolen, used by other members of the household.

        v. Can impair cognitive performance.

      e. Contraindications

         i. History of drug abuse or drug-seeking behavior.

        ii. Occupation requiring optimal cognitive performance: driver, pilot, military, etc. This is a relative contraindication, because, for example, severe, chronic sleep deprivation due to pain that is unrelieved by any other medication may impair cognitive performance even more.

(5) Short-acting narcotics

      a. Oxycodone 5 mg tabs 1 to 2 po q 4 hrs prn severe headache.

      b. Percocet (oxycodone 5 mg/acetaminophen 325 mg) 1 to 2 tabs po q 4 hrs prn severe headache, typically no more than 6 pills per 24 hours, absolute maximum 12 tabs per 24 hours (4000 mg total acetaminophen from all sources).

      c. Many alternatives, including combinations of narcotics and other analgesics.

      d. Advantages

         i. Very effective in the short term.

        ii. Some anxiety relieving effects as well.

       iii. Rapidly reversible with naloxone in case of overdose.

      e. Disadvantages

         i. Habit forming, risk of worsening the opioid epidemic.

    ii. Tolerance develops.

    iii. Street value: high risk of being lost, stolen, used by other members of the household.

    iv. Can impair cognitive performance.

    v. Constipation: often a good idea to offer Colace 100 mg po bid and Senna 25 mg po bid along with the narcotic.

    vi. Written signature and Drug Enforcement Agency (DEA) number required for each prescription. Cannot be prescribed by independent nurse practitioners.

  f. Contraindications

    i. History of drug abuse or drug-seeking behavior.

    ii. Pulmonary disorders that would increase risk adverse outcome in case of respiratory depression.

    iii. Occupation requiring optimal cognitive performance: driver, pilot, military, etc. This is a relative contraindication, because, for example, severe, chronic sleep deprivation due to pain that is unrelieved by any other medication may impair cognitive performance even more.

(6) Calcitonin Gene Related Peptide (CGRP) pathway mediations. This class of medications is just becoming available. Little is known about the effects of these medications on post-traumatic headache, though there is some evidence from animal models that CGRP is involved in the pathophysiology of headache after injury. They seem to be very safe and are worth a try.

(7) Transcranial Magnetic Stimulation. A hand-held transcranial magnetic stimulation device called HandSpring TMS is approved by the Food and Drug Administration (FDA) for acute treatment of migraine. Little is known about its effect in concussion-related headaches.

Migraine Prophylaxis

Who: 3 or more impairing headaches per week, *or* any frequency of truly disabling headaches that don't respond well to "as needed" medications.

When: Relatively early. If the patient is still having headaches more than 2 weeks after concussion, consider starting prophylactic medication.

Why: "As needed" pain medications in high doses may lose effectiveness over time, cause side effects, and increase the risk of developing medication overuse headaches.

How: Mostly just like treating regular migraine, with a few exceptions (see discussion later in this chapter). In general, concussion patients can often be more sensitive to side effects than others and do better with slower titration.

There isn't much difference in overall efficacy between medications *on average*, but every patient is different, and it can take some trial and error to find the right treatment for each individual patient.

Consider using a quantitative scale such as the Headache Impact Test (HIT6) or Migraine Disability Assessment Test (MIDAS) at each visit to assess whether the prophylaxis is working.

(1) Amitriptyline (Elavil): Often a first choice because there are decades of experience in concussion patients.
   a. Initial dosing: 25 mg po qhs
   b. Alternative dosing: 12.5 mg qhs x 7 days, then 25 mg po qhs for patients who may be very sensitive to the side effects, for example, smaller patients, patients taking other sleep-promoting medications, patients with constipation at baseline.
   c. Alternative dosing: 25 mg po qhs x 7 days, then 50 mg po qhs for larger patients.
   d. Time to effect 4 to 6 weeks
   e. Monitoring: typically none needed.

   f. Frequency of dose adjustment: typically 4 to 6 weeks

   g. Maximum effective dose rarely more than 100 mg.

   h. What to expect: 50% reduction in frequency, or severity or both.

   i. Advantages

      i. Works especially well in kids and young adults.

      ii. Helps with insomnia. A "2 for 1" for some patients.

      iii. Used as an antidepressant (often at higher doses), which is useful to mention for "vitamin P" effect.

      iv. Inexpensive

   j. Disadvantages

      i. Anticholinergic side effects leading to early morning fatigue, dry mouth, constipation, etc. Warn patients about this in advance.

      ii. A small worsening of cognitive function in some sensitive patients. Watch carefully for this in older patients and switch meds if the risk–benefit relationship isn't worth it.

      iii. Some minor weight gain. Preempt this with advice about diet and exercise.

(2) Topiramate (Topamax)

   a. Dosing 25 mg po qd (any time of day)

   b. Alternative dosing: 12.5 mg po qd x 1 week, then 25 mg po qd. *It can be a good idea to start low and titrate slowly if concerned about cognitive side effects.*

   c. Alternative dosing: 25 mg po qd x 1 week, then 25 mg po bid

   d. Time to effect: 4 to 6 weeks

   e. Monitoring: typically none needed.

   f. Adjust dose for renal function.

   g. Frequency of dose adjustment: typically 4 to 6 weeks

   h. Maximum effective dose rarely more than 100 mg bid.

   i. What to expect: 50% or greater reduction in frequency, or severity, or both.

   j. Advantages

        i. Probably the most effective migraine prophylactic medication overall.

        ii. Some weight loss due to appetite suppression.

   k. Disadvantages

        i. Some cognitive side effects, especially word finding and speed of processing (nickname "dope-a-max"). This makes topiramate relatively less useful for concussion patients than for patients with migraine in other settings. Still worth it for many concussion patients.

        ii. Risk of kidney stones. Counsel patients to stay well hydrated.

        iii. Annoying carbonic anhydrase effect (tingling extremities, odd taste of carbonated drinks)

        iv. Some weight loss due to appetite suppression.

(3) Botulinum Toxin

   a. Dosing: 155 to 200 units injected into 31 sites around the head and neck every 12 weeks.

   b. Time to effect: within 4 weeks

   c. Monitoring: facial weakness, rare swallowing difficulties.

   d. Advantages: Can be effective when medications are not. We are often prescribing botulinum toxin after 2 failed medications. Very well tolerated.

   e. Disadvantages: Expensive, requires a skilled provider to administer.

(4) Propranolol (Inderal)

   a. Dosing 40 mg po TID

   b. Alternative dosing: 20 mg po TID x 7 days, then 40 mg po TID when there are specific concerns about side effects.

   c. Alternative dosing: 40 mg po TID x 7 days, then 80 mg po TID when a more substantial beta blocker effect is desired (e.g., coronary artery disease, poorly controlled hypertension).

   d. Time to effect: 4 to 6 weeks

e. Monitoring: blood pressure and heart rate weekly until dose is stable for 4 to 6 weeks.

f. Frequency of dose adjustment: typically 4 to 6 weeks

g. Maximum effective dose rarely more than 320 mg per day.

h. What to expect: 50% reduction in frequency, or severity, or both.

i. Advantages:

   i. Mood stabilizer in the setting of traumatic brain injury (Not under other circumstances. This is a difference between concussion-related migraine and migraine in other settings).

   ii. "2 for 1" in patients with coexisting coronary artery disease or uncontrolled hypertension.

   iii. Inexpensive

j. Disadvantages:

   i. Symptomatic bradycardia and orthostatic hypotension. Warn patients about this.

   ii. Can impair athletic performance.

   iii. Can worsen fatigue.

   iv. Can worsen major depression.

   v. Can worsen asthma.

   vi. Can cause sexual dysfunction.

   vii. Inconvenient to take TID. Switch to long-acting once-daily formulation when dose is stabilized.

(5) Verapamil (Calan, others)

a. Dosing: 40 mg po TID

b. Alternative dosing: 20 mg po TID x 7 days, then 40 mg po TID when there are specific concerns about side effects.

c. Alternative dosing: 40 mg po TID x 7 days, then 80 mg po TID when a more substantial calcium blocker effect is desired (e.g., poorly controlled hypertension).

d. Time to effect: 4 to 6 weeks

e. Monitoring: blood pressure and heart rate weekly until dose is stable for 4 to 6 weeks.

f. Frequency of dose adjustment: typically 4 to 6 weeks
g. Maximum effective dose rarely more than 320 mg per day.
h. What to expect: 50% reduction in frequency, or severity, or both.
i. Advantages:
   i. "2 for 1" in patients with coexisting uncontrolled hypertension.
   ii. Inexpensive
j. Disadvantages:
   i. Symptomatic bradycardia and hypotension. Warn patients about this.
   ii. Constipation
   iii. Can impair athletic performance.
   iv. Inconvenient to take TID. Switch to long-acting once-daily formulation when dose is stabilized.

(6) Extended release divalproex (Depakote ER)
a. Initial dosing: 500 mg po qhs
b. Alternative dosing for refractory very severe migraines or medication overuse headache: Valproic acid 20 mg/kg intravenous loading dose (1000 to 2000 mg for most people), then 10 mg/kg iv bid, adjusting dose each day until headache relieved or development of unacceptable side effects. Then 500 mg po qhs after hospital discharge.
c. Time to effect: 4 to 6 weeks for initial po dosing. 1 to 3 days for intravenous dosing.
d. Monitoring: Complete blood count and comprehensive metabolic panel before starting the medication for a baseline, then 4 to 6 weeks after each dosage adjustment, then yearly while on stable doses.
e. Frequency of dose adjustment: typically 4 to 6 weeks
f. Maximum effective dose rarely more than 2000 mg per day.
g. What to expect: 50% reduction in frequency, or severity or both.

    h. Advantages:
- i. Mood stabilizer, "2 for 1" in patients with coexisting mood instability or bipolar disorder.
- ii. Antiepileptic, "2 for 1" in patients with coexisting seizure disorder.
- iii. Helps with insomnia. A "2 for 1" for some patients.
- iv. Available intravenously for a rapid load.

    i. Disadvantages:
- i. Cognitive impairment, especially memory and processing speed.
- ii. Fatigue during the day.
- iii. Often substantial weight gain. Critical to implement diet and exercise regimen immediately.
- iv. Rare liver and bone marrow toxicity. Monitor carefully and switch to another agent if elevated aspartate aminotransferase (AST), alanine aminotransferase (ALT), or if reduced white blood cell (WBC) or platelet count.
- v. High risk of fetal malformations. Contraindicated in pregnancy and relatively contraindicated in women of childbearing potential.

(7) Other medications: duloxetine (Cymbalta), fluoxetine (Prozac), gabapentin (Neurontin), levetiracetam (Keppra), magnesium, memantine (Namenda), riboflavin, olanzapine (Zyprexa), paroxetine (Paxil), pregabalin (Lyrica), zonisamide (Zonegran), etc., etc., etc. Many other medications have been used for migraine prophylaxis, with little information about their effect in the setting of concussion.

(8) Calcitonin Gene Related Peptide (CGRP) pathway medications: This class of medications is just becoming available. Little is known about the effects of these medications on post-traumatic headache, though clinical trials are on-going. They seem to be very safe and are worth a try.

(9) Cognitive Behavioral Therapy. Importantly, cognitive behavioral therapy may reduce pain interference with activities,

in addition to the pain itself. This type of treatment may be appealing for those who don't want to or cannot take medications. In adolescents with chronic migraine, cognitive behavioral therapy plus amitriptyline reduced migraine headache more than headache education plus amitriptyline (Powers et al., JAMA, 2013). The effects in concussion patients and other age groups are not known but may be similar.

(10) Repetitive Transcranial Magnetic Stimulation. This type of treatment may also be appealing for those who don't want to or cannot take medications. Although it is FDA-approved for depression, it is not widely available as a treatment for headache and would usually not be covered by insurance at present. It's worth considering in patients who have not benefited from other treatments. The authors of a recent pilot study reported that repeated stimulation of the left motor cortex over 4 sessions decreased persistent and debilitating headaches in traumatic brain injury patients (Leung et al., Neuromodulation, 2016). Transcranial Magnetic Stimulation can cause seizures in susceptible individuals, but it is generally felt to be safe in most concussion patients. It is FDA-approved for treatment-resistant depression. Dorsolateral prefrontal cortex stimulation was reported to alleviate headaches and modestly improve depressive symptoms in concussive traumatic brain injury (TBI) patients (Leung et al., Neuromodulation, 2018).

Acute Neuralgia /Neuropathic Pain Treatment

(1) Carbamazepine (Tegretol) 200 to 400 mg po immediately on onset of pain. It does not need to be taken regularly (unlike antiepileptic use). Max 2000 mg per day.
   a. Advantages: most effective, inexpensive. Response to carbamazepine can help with diagnosis.

      b. Disadvantages: lots of drug–drug interactions, some side effects if used frequently.

      c. Dose-limiting side effects include somnolence, dizziness, and nausea.

      d. If using frequently, check sodium levels and complete blood count (CBC).

(2) Oxcarbazepine (Trileptal): 150 to 600 mg po immediately on onset of pain. Max 1200 mg per day.

      a. Advantages: fewer side effects and fewer drug–drug interactions than carbamazepine.

      b. Disadvantages: more expensive, not always covered by insurance.

(3) Gabapentin (Neurontin) 300 to 1200 mg po immediately on onset of pain., Max 3600 mg per day.

      a. Advantage: very few side effects (mainly somnolence) or drug–drug interactions.

      b. Disadvantages: not very effective for severe pain. Not really even clear if it is better than placebo.

(4) Pregabalin (Lyrica) 50 to 100 mg po immediately on onset of pain. Max 200 mg per day.

      a. More effective than gabapentin.

      b. More somnolence.

      c. Some risk of thrombocytopenia and renal impairment. Check platelets and creatinine yearly if using chronically.

(5) Amitriptyline (Elavil) prophylaxis

      a. Initial dosing: 25 mg po qhs

      b. Alternative dosing: 12.5 mg qhs x 7 days, then 25 mg po qhs.

      c. Alternative dosing: 25 mg po qhs x 7 days, then 50 mg po qhs.

      d. Time to effect: 4 to 6 weeks

      e. Monitoring: typically none needed.

      f. Frequency of dose adjustment: typically 4 to 6 weeks.

      g. Advantages

         i. Works especially well in kids and young adults.

         ii. Helps with insomnia. A "2 for 1" for some patients.

      iii. Used as an antidepressant (at much higher doses), which is useful to mention for vitamin P effect.

      iv. Inexpensive

  h. Disadvantages

      i. Anticholinergic side effects leading to early morning fatigue, dry mouth, etc. Warn patients about this in advance.

      ii. A small worsening of cognitive function in some sensitive patients. Watch carefully for this in older patients and switch meds if the risk–benefit relationship isn't worth it.

      iii. Some minor weight gain. Preempt this with advice about diet and exercise.

Acute Tension Headache Treatment

(1) Ibuprofen (Motrin and many others) 400 to 800 mg po q 8 hours as needed.

  a. Not in patients with renal impairment.

  b. Not in certain postoperative patients.

  c. Not in patients with thrombocytopenia.

  d. For more than 24 hours, add GI prophylaxis.

(2) Naproxen (Aleve and others) 220 to 550 mg po q 12 hours as needed.

  a. Not in patients with renal impairment.

  b. Not in certain postoperative patients.

  c. Not in patients with thrombocytopenia.

  d. For more than 24 hours, add GI prophylaxis.

(3) Acetaminophen (Tylenol) 500 to 1000 mg po q 4 to 6 hours as needed, Max 4000 mg per 24 hours.

  a. Not in patients with liver failure.

(4) Narcotics rarely, if ever. Consider if and only if the headaches are severe, impairing, and refractory to other medications. This is atypical for uncomplicated tension headache. If the patient requires narcotics for tension headache, this should

prompt a re-evaluation of the diagnosis and a careful assessment of social factors (Drug seeking? Previous narcotic addiction? Selling or trading medication?).

Musculoskeletal Neck Pain

(1) Start with rest and over-the-counter analgesics for 1 week.
   a. Acetaminophen (Tylenol and many others) 1000 mg up to 4 times per day.
      i. Contraindicated in liver failure or active liver disease.
   b. Ibuprofen (Motrin and many others) 600 mg up to 3 times per day.
      i. Contraindicated in renal failure, NSAID-related GI bleeding, and after some long-bone fractures or orthopedic surgeries.
(2) If 1 week of rest and over-the counter analgesics are not effective, consider prescribing a soft collar to relieve pressure on the neck and allow muscles to heal over 4 to 12 weeks.
   a. The patient should not exercise the neck while there is still pain.
   b. After the pain has subsided, then the patient should be referred for physical therapy to gently restart strengthening the neck muscles. There will be some deconditioning while the collar is on, so if the patient goes straight back to full exertion, there is risk of reinjuring the neck. There is evidence from randomized trials that early cervical spine and vestibular physical therapy leads to faster return to sport participation in young athletes with persistent symptoms of dizziness, neck pain, and/or headaches (Schneider et al., British Journal of Sports Medicine, 2014).
(3) Consider acupuncture treatment. Acupuncture was used effectively in the acute phase after concussion by U.S. military treatment providers in Afghanistan, especially when there were contraindications to medications with potential

cognitive side effects. In a small randomized controlled trial performed in military service members with TBI after return to the United States, both auricular acupuncture and traditional Chinese acupuncture reduced headache severity more than usual care when given in 10 sessions over 6 weeks (Jonas et al., Medical Acupuncture, 2016).

(4) Generally avoid sedating medications such as methocarbamol (Robaxin), metaxalone (Skelaxin), and cyclobenzaprine (Flexeril) in the setting of concussion, because these medications can cause cognitive impairment.

Medication overuse headaches: *Consider admitting patients with medication overuse headaches to the hospital* for supervised withdrawal and intravenous dihydroergotamine (D.H.E. 45), valproate (Depacon), or ziprasidone (Geodon). *In many cases, nothing will work well on an outpatient basis.* Better to do this sooner rather than later, so that the patient can move on to rehabilitation. Usually, this should be handled by a Neurology or Anesthesia hospital service with experience in medication overuse headache treatment. The specific details are beyond the scope of this manual. Please see additional references (e.g., *Wolff's Headache and Other Head Pain*, Chapter 11) for details.

Acute Cluster Headache Treatment

(1) Inhale 100% oxygen through a mask at > 7 liters per minute. An optimal choice as these headaches come on suddenly. Caution in patients with chronic obstructive pulmonary disease (COPD) who should be monitored due to risk of hypoventilation.

(2) Triptans, especially fast-acting forms: injection and nasal spray. Same contraindications as in migraine.

(3) Dihydroergotamine (DHE) intravenous. Risk of nausea. Same contraindications as for triptans.

(4) Octreotide injectable. No data in the setting of brain injury.

8

Sleep Disruption

You have to get this right; everything else hinges on it. Patients will get worse over time, not better, if they accumulate more and more sleep deficit from chronic insomnia. See Figure 8.1.

The hierarchy for sleep is as follows: Best is good-quality natural sleep, second best is pharmacologically enhanced good-quality sleep, worst is insufficient or poor-quality sleep.

There are 3 basic types of insomnia: trouble getting to sleep, trouble staying asleep, and waking up too early without being able to get back to sleep. Patients can have more than one type. Ask the patient and the collateral source. If there are doubts, have a sleep study performed. Patients can be remarkably unreliable historians with regard to their own sleeping habits.

The tools

(1) Pain control. Treat pain aggressively, both headaches and other types of pain. No one can sleep if they are in too much pain. Even pain that is tolerable during the daytime can impair sleep at nighttime. Traumatic brain injury has been reported to increase pain symptoms in other parts of the body, such as from a limb fracture (Jodoin et al., Injury, 2017).

   a. Physical therapy can be very helpful for back and neck pain. Make sure the therapist understands that pain control is the priority, rather than, for example, cardiovascular fitness, range of motion, or improved balance.

   b. Over-the-counter analgesics and nonsteroidal anti-inflammatory medications.

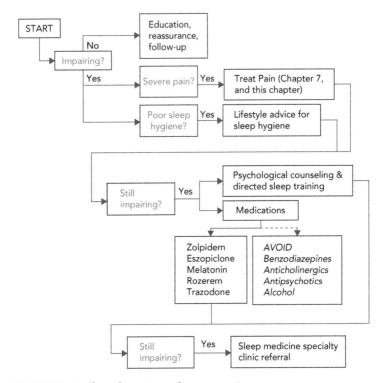

FIGURE 8.1 Sleep disruption after concussion.

  i. Ibuprofen (Motrin, others) 800 mg with a light snack each night before bedtime, as long as there is not renal failure or other contraindication.
  ii. Acetaminophen (Tylenol, others) 1000 mg each night before bedtime, as long as there is no liver failure or other contraindication.
  iii. Celecoxib (Celebrex) 100 to 200 mg each night before bedtime.
  c. A neuropathic pain medication, which may also have some sedating effects.
  i. Amitriptyline (Elavil) 25 mg each night x 1 week, then 50 mg each night.
  ii. Pregabalin (Lyrica) 50 mg each night.

       iii. Gabapentin (Neurontin) 300 mg each night x 1 week, then 800 mg each night.

   d. A narcotic or other short-term use pain medication only in the most severe cases. Examples:

       i. Tramadol (Ultram) 50 mg each night for 1 week, then 100 each night, as long as there is no seizure disorder.

       ii. Oxycodone 5 mg each night for 1 week, then 10 mg each night, as long as there is no history of narcotic misuse or dependence.

   e. A patient with serious chronic pain that doesn't respond to these interventions probably needs to be seen by a specialist in pain management who can safely perform targeted interventional procedures, prescribe long-active narcotics, and potentially even recommend implantation of an intrathecal delivery device.

      Consider starting with both (a) and (b) together, then others later if the first steps don't solve the problem.

(2) Cognitive behavioral therapy for insomnia. Cognitive behavioral therapy for insomnia has the strongest evidence base for efficacy, and it is the recommended first-line treatment. The authors of a recently published pilot study reported that 8 sessions of cognitive behavioral therapy for insomnia adapted for a mixed group of traumatic brain injury (TBI) patients was more effective than treatment as usual, with benefits on sleep quality, fatigue, and depression symptoms (Nguyen et al., Archives of Physical Medicine and Rehabilitation, 2017). Refer to a psychologist or other therapist with specific training in management of insomnia. Treatment may include mixed modalities such as mindfulness-based therapy and relaxation therapy, though other modalities do not have as strong an evidence base as cognitive behavioral therapy. Telephone-based cognitive behavioral therapy and Internet-based cognitive behavioral therapy are excellent alternatives to in-person therapy. If none of these options

are available, or the patient cannot afford them, consider offering the following suggestions:

a. Get at least 30 minutes of very bright light exposure each morning. This helps reset the patient's natural circadian clock. The best sources are sunlight, or a special lamp of the type used to treat seasonal affective disorders, which has lots of blue light. Regular indoor lights are not sufficient.

b. No caffeine or other stimulants for 8 hours before bedtime. Ask specifically about coffee, tea, soda, energy drinks, supplements, migraine medications, and herbal or traditional remedies. Not all patients realize that some of these have caffeine in them.

c. Restrict sleep in the daytime, which will increase sleep drive at night.

d. No heavy meals or spicy foods for 3 hours before bedtime.

e. Wind down for 1 hour before bedtime. No loud music, violent movies, exciting video games, or anything except for quiet, calm music and light reading for 1 hour before bedtime.

f. Go to bed at the same time every night.

g. Bedroom should be cool, dark, quiet, and comfortable. Adjust the thermostat, use dark blinds, turn off the music and the TV (there are some cultural differences that can be challenging), and maybe get a new mattress.

h. Write down your "to do" list for tomorrow before bed so you don't dwell on it.

i. Learn progressive muscle relaxation and practice it every night.

j. Visualize a quiet, calm, and peaceful place where you have slept really well in the past.

k. Don't use the bed for anything except sleep and intercourse. No reading, TV, videogames, etc. in bed.

l. If you don't fall asleep within 30 minutes, get up, go into another quiet, cool room, and read or listen to relaxing music until you get sleepy, then go back to bed.

(3) Sleep medications
   a. Melatonin 2 to 5 mg each night. Melatonin is a nat-
      ural substance produced by the body that rises at night
      in a circadian fashion. Melatonin is very safe and avail-
      able over the counter. A randomized controlled trial
      performed mainly in severe TBI patients demonstrated
      some benefit of 2 mg sustained-release melatonin taken
      2 hours before bedtime on sleep quality, daytime fatigue,
      and anxiety (Grima et al., BMC Medicine, 2018). Severe
      TBI patients may have more disrupted circadian rhythms
      than concussion patients; the effects seem to be more
      modest in concussion patients.
   b. Regular zolpidem (Ambien) 5 to 10 mg each night. This
      is good for either trouble falling asleep or trouble with
      mid-sleep awakening. It lasts ~4 hours, so tell the patient
      to take it only when he or she has at least 4 hours be-
      fore needing to get up. Although it is only approved by
      the U.S. Food and Drug Administration (FDA) for short-
      term use, there has been a great deal of experience with
      patients taking it for years without substantial long-term
      concerns. It loses efficacy, however, if taken every night.
      It works better when used relatively infrequently. Warn
      the patient and collateral source about the risk of odd
      behaviors such as sleep–eating. This does not seem to
      be any more common in concussion patients than in the
      general public; it is quite rare.
   c. Eszopiclone (Lunesta) 2 to 3 mg each night. This is good
      for trouble falling asleep and staying asleep. It lasts ~6
      hours, so it is usually not a good choice for mid-sleep
      awakening. Again, although it is only indicated for short-
      term use, there has been a great deal of experience with
      patients taking it for years without substantial long-term
      concerns. Again, it loses efficacy if taken every night. It
      works better when used relatively infrequently.
   d. Zolpidem Extended Release (Ambien CR) 6.25 to 12.5 mg
      each night. This is good for trouble falling asleep, staying

asleep, and waking up too early. It lasts ~8 hours, so it should not be used by people who have to do important tasks immediately upon awakening.

e. Ramelteon (Rozerem) 8 mg each night. This is a very safe medication that acts as a melatonin agonist. Like melatonin itself, its effects are modest, but it can be worth trying when there are contraindications to other medications.

f. Trazodone 50 to 100 mg each night. This medication has the advantage of also being an antidepressant. However, it commonly causes patients to feel groggy or hung over the next morning. Although commonly used in concussion patients, other medications may be preferred when the goal is to optimize cognitive recovery.

(4) Stop other medications that can impair recovery and cognitive function.

a. *Avoid* short-acting benzodiazepines such as alprazolam (Xanax), lorazepam (Ativan), and diazepam (Valium). These are very habit forming, impair cognitive function, and not a good idea unless they are being used to treat severe anxiety.

b. *Avoid* anticholinergic medications such as diphenhydramine (Benadryl and many others). These impair cognitive function. They are the main ingredient in most over-the-counter sleep aides, such as Unisom, Tylenol-PM, and Simply Sleep and are also found in cold remedies such as Contac, Theraflu, Benadryl Cold, and Sudafed Night-time. Consider telling the patient that even though these are sold over the counter, they are less safe in the setting of concussion than some prescription medications.

c. *Avoid* antipsychotics like quetiapine (Seroquel) and risperidone (Risperdal) unless they are being used to treat psychosis, obsessive compulsive disorder, or another serious psychiatric condition. These impair cognitive function and often cause weight gain.

    d. *Avoid* using alcohol as a sleep aide. Alcohol markedly impairs the recovery of the brain from injury and interferes with the effects of many other medications. Sometimes patients don't like this. Tell them kindly your job is not to tell them what they want to hear, but to give them best medical advice.

(5) Refer to a sleep medicine clinic for a consultation and a formal sleep study. Sometimes restless leg syndrome, sleep apnea, or parasomnias can be causes of apparent insomnia, even if the patient and collateral source are not aware of them.

These tools are not necessarily listed in order of priority. Every patient is different. Choose from among them like a menu. If the patient can get right into cognitive behavioral therapy for insomnia and benefit quickly, this is optimal. If not, it is OK to start with a medication with the idea that it later can be weaned off of once patients have learned from cognitive behavioral therapy, and their pain control strategy is in place.

Consider using a quantitative tool such as the Insomnia Severity Index (https://www.myhealth.va.gov/mhv-portal-web/insomnia-severity-index) at each visit to assess whether the interventions are working.

9

Attention Deficit

Many concussion patients complain of problems with memory, usually short-term memory. Upon taking a careful history and upon examination, however, it is more common for them to have deficits in attention rather than memory per se (see Table 9.1). In everyday life, attention deficit manifests in part as forgetfulness for details: "He went to the store and forgot to get the milk" or "I constantly forget where I left my keys." Most people don't clearly differentiate between attention and memory. It is important to distinguish, because attention and memory are optimally treated differently, or if both are significant concerns, both should be treated.

The good news is that attention deficit is very treatable, whereas most types of true memory failure (amnesic syndromes) are not particularly treatable (See Chapter 18). Furthermore, many patients, perhaps a higher proportion of concussion patients than the general population, have a history of attention deficit prior to injury. In fact, attention deficit may be a risk factor for concussion. So after concussion, the underlying treated or compensated attention deficit can be exacerbated. This is not always the case—there are plenty of concussion patients with new onset attention deficit who did not have any attention deficit before injury, so the absence of a history of attention deficit should not influence the diagnostic assessment.

There are many options for managing attention deficit, divided here into "Aggressive, "Moderate," and "Conservative" approaches. Mainly these differ with regard to use of neuropsychological testing and treatment with stimulants, but there are other management choices as well (see Table 9.2). The treating provider, the patient, and the patient's family all have to be comfortable with the approach chosen.

TABLE 9.1 How Do You Tell the Difference between Problems with Memory versus Attention?

	Memory Impairment	*Attention Deficit*
Formal Neuropsychological Testing	Impairment on quantitative and standardized tests of immediate and delayed recall.	Impairment on quantitative and standardized tests of sustained vigilance, reaction times, and working memory.
Bedside Cognitive Testing	Errors on informal tests of immediate and delayed recall	Errors on informal tests of sustained attention to task
Everyday Life Symptoms	Getting lost. Losing things permanently and not being aware of the loss. Forgetting important people, places, and events. Difficulty learning new facts or new skills.	Misplacing things but finding them again later. Trouble staying focused on tasks. Trouble restarting a task after an interruption.
Source	Patient may or may not be aware of the deficits. Often more troubling to others than to the patient.	Concerning to both patient and others

The approach taken also depends on the timing relative to the concussion. Attention deficits in the first 1 to 2 weeks after concussion that are resolving do not warrant an aggressive approach. Natural recovery will be enough. However, attention deficit that

TABLE 9.2 Approaches to Treatment of Attention Deficit after Concussion

	Aggressive	Moderate	Conservative
Treatment for Insomnia	Yes	Yes	Yes
Treatment for Migraine	Yes	Yes	Yes
Alcohol	Stop completely	Limit	Limit
Cardiovascular Exercise	Prescribe	Prescribe	Recommend
Cognitive Rehabilitation	Prescribe	Prescribe	Prescribe if neuropsychological testing indicates attention deficit
Stimulants	Prescribe	Prescribe if other approaches not successful and neuropsychological testing indicates attention deficit	None unless pre-injury attention deficit and no contraindications.
Acetylcholinesterase Inhibitors	Prescribe if stimulants not fully effective	Prescribe if stimulants not fully effective	None unless indicated for dementia
Caffeine	Prescribe if stimulants contraindicated	Recommend if stimulants contraindicated	No recommendation
Refined Sugar	Reduce or eliminate	Recommend healthy diet	Recommend healthy diet
Passive Activities	Reduce or eliminate	No recommendation	No recommendation

is not improving several months after concussion is not likely to resolve on its own, and active treatment is appropriate. See Figure 9.1.

Aggressive: Treat the attention deficit based on *symptoms* reported by the patient *or the collateral source.* This does not require neuropsychological testing evidence of attention deficit. Neuropsychological testing can be helpful, but if the patient can't function in the real world and their neuropsychological testing is normal, they still can't function in the real world. Concussion patients can deteriorate when distracted, and be less effective at eliminating distractions, so the patients' performance in a quiet room without distractions may

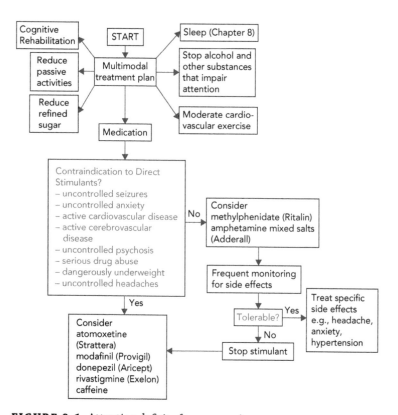

FIGURE 9.1 Attention deficit after concussion.

not be indicative of real world performance. Likewise, performance on emotionally neutral attention tasks may not reflect performance on emotionally charged attention tasks. This doesn't mean that all of the impairments are due to depression or emotional problems. In the real world, it may not be possible to fully separate attention from emotional regulation. Furthermore, migraine aura or cogniphobia during testing may cause erratic or hard-to-interpret neuropsychological test results. Thus, even without solid neuropsychological testing evidence for attention deficit, the aggressive interventions for attention still help many patients function in the real world and improve their quality of life after concussion.

Moderate: No stimulants unless the patient has documented attention deficit on formal neuropsychological testing. Consider starting with cognitive rehabilitation, treatment of insomnia, and cessation of cognitively impairing substances such as alcohol and prescription medications. Then, if the patient does not improve, order formal neuropsychological testing and consider additional treatment options including stimulants, if there is evidence of attention deficit and no contraindication.

Conservative: No stimulants unless the patient has a preinjury history of attention deficit disorder and absolutely no vascular risk factors (age < 40, no high blood pressure, no diabetes, nonsmoker, no high cholesterol, no family history of early heart disease).

Specific Treatments for Attention Deficit

(1) *Treatment for insomnia:* No one can concentrate properly without a good night's sleep. Sometimes this is the only intervention necessary to treat attention deficit after concussion. The most aggressive intervention plans may include a stimulant in the daytime, then a sleep-promoting therapy or medication at bedtime (see Chapter 8).

(2) *Treatment for migraine:* Migraine can cause cognitive impairment during the aura phase as well as during the headache itself. Cogniphobia ("my head hurts worse when

I concentrate") makes real-world cognitive performance worse. After migraines have resolved, patients are often very fatigued, limiting their cognitive activities (see Chapter 7).

(3) *Stop alcohol:* Even a small amount of alcohol can impair attention in concussion patients. They often report being more sensitive to the cognitive effects of alcohol than prior to injury, even if they don't feel "buzzed" or drunk at all. Consider recommending that the patient not drink any alcohol at all for the first 12 months to allow the best chance for a full recovery. It is not necessary to be dogmatic about this. A toast at a wedding or a single drink on a Friday night isn't going to undo everything. There is a lot of resistance to this—many patients either don't tell the doctor how much they are drinking or don't acknowledge its effects. Sometimes a family member will bring this to attention by phone or e-mail after the initial visit. The job of the provider isn't to tell patients what they want to hear, it is to give them the best medical advice. Peer pressure can be a big problem. Patients who know they should stop drinking after concussion but can't resist the peer pressure may need a face-saving way to do the right thing. Consider writing on a prescription pad, "No alcohol at all for any reason" and tell patients that they can tell their friends a white lie—"I am on a med for my headaches that won't work if I drink." This can be quite successful if done sensitively. Importantly, inquire about alcohol, marijuana, and other illicit drugs sensitively and repeatedly. It is common for the real story to come from the collateral source or from the patient at follow-up, rather than on the initial visit. It's also especially sensitive for military service members (see Chapter 37).

(4) *Cardiovascular exercise:* Consider writing a prescription for "Moderately intense cardiovascular exercise 30 to 60 minutes per day, 6 days per week *whether you feel like it or not.*" It may be necessary to refer to physical therapy (PT) with specific instructions to design an exercise program for the patient that he can tolerate for the rest of his life. A good

personal trainer is helpful for motivation, variety, and good technique if the patient can afford it. Again, it is helpful to give the trainer explicit instructions. For attention deficit after concussion, the treatment should be sustained cardiovascular exercise, even if the patient says she wants to build muscle, improve athletic performance, etc.

(5) *Cognitive rehabilitation:* Based on symptoms reported by the patient *or the collateral source,* consider prescribing speech therapy (ST), occupational therapy (OT), and treatment at an occupational performance center if available. This does not require neuropsychological testing-based evidence for attention deficit. The treating provider should explicitly direct the therapists to focus treatment on attention training. This training has many forms, but usually consists of exercises done initially in a nondistracting environment, then gradually increasing the level of distraction during the exercises. Often, common real-world distractions will be brought in—a cell phone that rings, a text message arriving, a person coming over to talk, etc. Then the therapist will direct the patient to get back to the task at hand and practice redirecting attention after interruption. Also, the therapist may give explicit instructions for how to reduce distractions: for example, turn off the TV, radio, and cell phone; avoid instant messaging or e-mail applications open on the computer; or go to a place like the library or a part of the house where there are fewer interruptions. Patients often resist these instructions because they may prefer their distractions to their actual work, but cognitive rehabilitation can be like "boot camp" for the brain. It isn't fun, but it makes you stronger. Appropriate cognitive rehabilitation combined with stimulants can be more beneficial than either therapy alone. For example, in a recent randomized controlled trial, a rehabilitation technique called Memory and Attention Adaptation Training paired with methylphenidate was shown to be more effective than Memory and Attention Adaptation Training plus placebo, and more

effective than an alternative technique called Attention Builders Training paired with methylphenidate (McDonald et al., Neuropharmacology, 2016).

(6) *Stimulants*: Stimulants are probably the single most effective pharmacological agent available to improve cognitive performance after concussion. When effective, patients describe the feeling as being "like a really good cup of coffee," "in the zone," or "back to almost normal for a few hours." Stimulants are prescribed frequently, despite the risks and the potential for abuse (see discussion later in this chapter 38). With these guidelines, they can be used safely, but this approach is sometimes considered more "aggressive" and may fall outside some providers' comfort levels.

a. *Absolute contraindications*:

  i. Uncontrolled seizure disorder. Treat the seizure disorder first. Stimulants will make it worse. Get a neurology consult right away if appropriate. It is sometimes safe to start stimulants after 6 months of seizure freedom. With this long-term goal, consider medications such as levetiracetam (Keppra), lamotrigine (Lamictal), and oxcarbazepine (Trileptal) that cause less impairment of attentional performance than other medications. Importantly, treatment with stimulants does not appear to increase the risk of seizures in patients with attention deficit who have not previously had seizures.

  ii. Uncontrolled panic attacks or dangerous anxiety disorder. Again, stimulants will make this worse. Get a psychiatry consult right away if appropriate. It is sometimes safe to start stimulants after 6 weeks of an anxiolytic medication and lifestyle modification. Somewhat counterintuitively, post-traumatic stress disorder (PTSD) does not seem to be a contraindication to stimulant use, and stimulants may even sometimes improve PTSD symptoms.

iii. Symptoms of active cardiovascular disease, such as "cardiac" chest pain, dyspnea on exertion, and markedly reduced exercise tolerance. This issue causes the most concern for many practitioners. Get a cardiology consult right away. Consider ordering an exercise echo cardiogram stress test. Note that cardiac risk factors alone (age, hypertension, diabetes, hypercholesterolemia, smoking, family history) are not absolute contraindications, but it is prudent to assess for cardiovascular disease before prescribing stimulants. It may be possible to start stimulants after risk factors have been adequately managed, but it is rarely if ever safe to prescribe stimulants in patients with active cardiovascular disease.

iv. Active cerebrovascular disease. A history of stroke, recent transient ischemic attack (TIA), or known cerebrovascular malformation. Get a neurology consult if the history or exam is not clear. Get a magnetic resonance angiogram (MRA) or computed tomography (CT) angiogram if you are not sure. It is rarely if ever safe to give stimulants to patients with aneurysms or arteriovenous malformations. Consult neurology or neurosurgery if the interpretation of the scan is not straightforward.

v. Active psychosis. Hallucinations or delusions can get worse with stimulants. Consult psychiatry if appropriate. It can be safe to prescribe a stimulant along with a small dose of an atypical antipsychotic in patients with relatively mild hallucinations or delusions that are not dangerous to themselves or others. It is rarely if ever safe, however, to use them in patients who are so out of touch with reality that they cannot be monitored for side effects reliably.

vi. A history of serious drug abuse or irresponsible criminal behavior. Stimulants have potential for abuse and have a street value. Take a collateral history in private. A patient interested in getting stimulants may tell you about symptoms that are consistent with attention deficit and deny any history of drug abuse or criminal behavior. A sensitive discussion with a mature and reliable collateral source (parent, spouse, employer, teacher) will usually get to the bottom of things. It may be possible to effectively treat former drug abusers with stimulants in a controlled setting. For example, a group home where the staff keeps the medications, dispenses them one at a time, and makes sure the patient actually swallows them.

vii. Dangerously underweight. Stimulants suppress the appetite, which can be a good thing for many patients, but can be dangerous. It is rarely if ever safe to prescribe stimulants to patients with active anorexia nervosa, cancer-related weight loss, or recent malnutrition. Once these issues have been resolved, it may be safe to treat with stimulants.

viii. Uncontrolled headaches. Migraine and tension headaches may become significantly worse with stimulants. It is sometimes safe to start stimulants after headaches have been relatively well controlled for several weeks. With this in mind, consider migraine prophylactic treatments that cause relatively little daytime impairment of attention, such as botulinum toxin, small doses of amitriptyline, verapamil, or propranolol.

b. *Specific medications*:

i. Methylphenidate (Ritalin): Consider starting with methylphenidate (Ritalin) because there is the most experience with it in the setting of traumatic brain injury, and it has the shortest half-life. If there are any problems, they usually won't last more than 3 to 4 hours. The effective dose varies widely among individuals. Sometimes 5 mg each morning and 5 mg each day at noon. Sometimes up to 20 mg three times a day. The clinical trials have typically used 0.3 mg/kg twice per day. It can be titrated up as fast as every 3 days with proper monitoring for side effects.

ii. Longer acting stimulants such as amphetamine mixed salts (Adderall, Adderall XR), Ritalin LA, etc. If a patient says, "I get a good effect from the Ritalin, but it wears off too soon and I crash," this may be an indication to switch to a longer acting medication. Overall, the risks and benefits are similar for all the medications in the class. For the longer acting agents, monitor for insomnia more carefully because this is more of a concern than for shorter acting methylphenidate (Ritalin).

iii. Methylphenidate transdermal (Daytrana patch). This can be very effective because of the smooth continuous delivery of methylphenidate for 9 hours.

iv. Mixed regimens: A larger dose of a long-acting medication in the morning and a small dose of regular short-acting methylphenidate in the mid-afternoon can be very effective for patients with severe attention deficit without causing insomnia.

v. Atomoxetine (Strattera): relatively weak effects. May be helpful as an adjunct when getting to the limits of tolerability of the real stimulants. Not typically a primary treatment.

c. *"How long will I be on this?"* Some people can stay on stimulants for decades. Others may only need them for a few months. As long as there are none of the contraindications listed above, stimulants can be used safely for decades. Reassess every 6 months: Tell the patient to stop taking the stimulant for 1 week and ask the collateral source what happened. It is OK to just stop stimulants—there is no need to taper. If patients get a lot worse, then clearly, they were still benefitting.

d. *How to avoid tolerance and reduce long-term adverse effects.* If the patient does need to take stimulants for more than 6 months, it is important to use them in a way so as to minimize the development of tolerance and make sure the patient continues to get appropriate benefit.

    i. Use 6 days per week rather than 7. Catch up on rest and light activities 1 day per week. Don't expect to do anything too important on the off day.

    ii. Use 51 weeks per year rather than 52. Take a true drug holiday, timed carefully to avoid problems with work or important cognitively engaging family activities. Sometimes the week between Christmas and New Year's works well, or a random week in the middle of the summer when nothing important is going on. Don't expect to do anything too difficult during the off week.

    iii. Cardiovascular exercise. This reduces anxiety, improves sleep, reduces cardiovascular and cerebrovascular risks, and may improve attention on its own. In the long-term, cardiovascular exercise is as important or more important that any medication. Consider asking the family and friends to get the patient out to exercise even when the patient doesn't feel like it. Recommend a personal trainer if the patient can afford one.

e. *The Rules.* Stimulant medications really work, and because they really work, they also have potential for abuse. A lot of providers are hesitant to prescribe stimulants because of issues of potential misuse. With strict adherence to Rules 1 to 4 below, there should be very few problems. Discuss the rules and ask the patient and collateral source to agree to them in writing before prescribing stimulants. Instruct the office staff about the rules, so that they can consistently enforce them for prescription refills (see Section III, Chapter 37).

    i. No abuse: "You cannot take more than prescribed or take them in any way that is not exactly as prescribed.

Call me or email me if you want to try something different."

ii. No sharing: "No one but you can take these. Don't even tell anyone you have them. Keep them in a place where no one else can get them, ideally in a locked cabinet."

iii. No selling: "I will fire you as a patient if you ever sell stimulants. That is a crime. You can go to jail. I know that they have a street value, but it just isn't worth it. Recovery from your concussion will help you have the best chance of getting a good job, and that will be worth a lot more money for you in the long term."

iv. No early refills: "If you lose a bottle of pills or run out early, I'm sorry but I will not provide any extra refills. If you have a police report documenting that they were stolen, I may make an exception."

f. *Careful monitoring for side effects.* This is important. Without careful monitoring for side effects, treatment with stimulants is more than aggressive, it is reckless. A lot of concussion patients are young and otherwise healthy and will not have any issues at all, but these medications when used appropriately can be safe and effective in more complex and older patients with careful monitoring.

i. Blood pressure and heart rate. Measure after each dose change *while patients have medication in their body.* A patient may have a normal blood pressure and heart rate before taking the medication or after it has worn off, but still have elevations in blood pressure and heart rate while on the drug. Consider obtaining a 9 AM check after an 8 AM dose. A primary doctor's office can do this and report back, or a nurse in the office can do this—these don't necessarily require a full follow-up visit. If there is a clear benefit of the stimulant, and the blood pressure and heart rate are elevated, consider treating with metoprolol, approximately 25 mg along with each 5 mg of methylphenidate. Metoprolol nicely balances the peripheral cardiovascular effects without blocking the central nervous system effects. Likewise, long-acting metoprolol (Toprol XL) balances the longer acting stimulants. Propranolol is not a good choice because it can block some of the central nervous system benefits of stimulants.

ii. Weight. Check the patient's weight 1 week after each dose change and once a month thereafter. Any undesired weight loss or more than 1 pound weight loss per week should trigger a re-evaluation. On the other hand, moderate weight loss can be a substantial benefit to some patients and encourage compliance with the rules.

iii. Take a focused interim history in person, by phone, or by e-mail. Ask both the patient and the collateral source about insomnia, anxiety, excessive weight loss, headaches, chest pain, exercise tolerance, psychosis, seizures, tremor, and new focal neurologic deficits that could represent a TIA or stroke. Consider seeing the patient in person for 5 minutes between regular patients if needed to assess.

(7) *Acetylcholinesterase inhibitors.* Donepezil (Aricept) and rivastigmine (Exelon) are commonly used in concussion patients. The effects on attention are more modest than stimulants. There is some evidence for benefit from clinical trials for both agents in more severe TBI patients. They are approved for patients with dementia, and in general they are well tolerated even by elderly patients.

a. Side effects that are most troubling:

i. GI upset. Usually minor and gets better within 1 to 2 weeks. If it is troubling, a dose reduction often will help: stop for 1 day, half dose (2.5 mg of donepezil) for 2 weeks then a slower titration (5 mg donepezil weeks 3 to 4), then full dose (10 mg donepezil) after that. Exelon patch has the added advantage of offering smooth delivery and may have reduced GI side effects as opposed to oral medication in concussion patients. Some patients may benefit from Exelon patch when they could not tolerate oral donepezil or oral rivastigmine.

ii. Headaches: These medications can exacerbate migraine and other headache disorders. Again, sometimes dose reduction and slow titration helps. But headache is often the limiting side effect for this class of medications in concussion patients. Consider treating headaches first before treating attention deficit. Stimulants, acetylcholinesterase inhibitors, and the intensive intellectual effort required for cognitive rehabilitation can make headaches worse.

iii. Seizures: These medications can reduce the seizure threshold in patients with known seizure disorder, but there are no reported cases of *new onset* seizures related to donepezil or rivastigmine in concussion patients.

(8) *Caffeine*. Prescribe a trial of a specific dose of caffeine: 100 mg first thing in the morning and 100 mg after lunch. Not more or less. Increase by 50 to 100 mg each week until there is a benefit or side effects. Usually 400 mg of caffeine per day is the maximum recommended dose, above which there is little additional benefit. For reference:

a. Regular coffee: 95 to 200 mg per 8 oz cup
b. Espresso coffee: 40 to 75 mg per 1 oz shot
c. Typical soft drinks: 30 to 50 mg per 12 oz can
d. Tea: 15 to 60 mg per 8 oz cup
e. Energy drinks (e.g., Red Bull, Rockstar, Monster): 50 to 200 mg per can
f. Caffeine-containing headache medications (e.g., Excedrin migraine): 65 mg per tablet
g. Over-the-counter caffeine tablets (e.g., NoDoz): up to 200 mg per tablet.

To avoid reduced effectiveness of caffeine or requirement for more and more, consider recommending caffeine use 6 days per week rather than 7 and 51 weeks per year rather than 52. Caffeine withdrawal headache can be a concern.

Contraindications to caffeine include tachycardia, severe anxiety, and certain cardiac arrhythmias. The most common side effects are insomnia, anxiety, worsening headache, and increased blood pressure.

Some patients with seizure disorder, drug abuse, poor appetite, or headaches can tolerate caffeine but cannot tolerate a stimulant.

(9) *Reduce refined sugar.* The scientific evidence for this is not strong, but in a subset of patients, reducing refined sugar may improve attentional performance. Usually this is in people who were not following a healthful diet prior to injury. A healthful normal diet is the goal. A nutrition consultation can be useful because many patients don't know what a healthful normal diet is. No special diets or food supplements have a proven benefit for attention deficit. Many of the "focus" supplements contain caffeine or other stimulants.

(10) *Reduce or eliminate passive activities.* Many people are habituated to passive activities such as watching TV/ movies/videos. But for the most highly motivated concussion patients who want to do everything they can to improve their attentional performance, reducing or eliminating passive activities may help. During down time, better to listen to music, go for a walk, engage in a hobby, do some light reading, or just rest quietly.

(11) *Other medications:* In our experience amantadine and modafinil are not particularly helpful for attention deficit in TBI patients. Modafinil (Provigil) does very little for attention. It is purely a wakefulness-enhancing drug and useful for somnolence but not for attention deficit. Amantadine is generally safe but doesn't have much benefit for attention. It may have some effects on fatigue, but these are

pretty modest compared to a real stimulant. A randomized controlled trial of amantadine demonstrated that there was no benefit in chronic TBI patients with a mixture of injury severities (Hammond et al., Journal of Neurotrauma, 2018).

Note, many of these treatments may improve cognitive performance in people without concussion as well, and in patients with nonconcussion-related attention deficit. It is possible to get the patient's attentional performance *better* than it was before injury using these methods, especially if they had an incompletely treated attention deficit prior to injury. This can sometimes blur the line between treatment and enhancement.

10

Mood Instability and Irritability

Often the complaint of mood instability and irritability comes from the collateral source: "He gets upset over things that never used to upset him"; "She's so moody"; "He's more quick tempered"; "One day she's fine and the next day she just won't get out of bed"; or "He cries whenever things don't go like we planned." All of these indicate that the patient doesn't have the same ability to keep the normal experiences of everyday life from affecting his or her outward expression of emotion. Many patients feel internally like they know these experiences shouldn't affect them, but they can't control themselves. Patients may report feeling "foolish," "weak" or "guilty." Sometimes dark thoughts, even suicidal or homicidal feelings or bizarre sexual urges, may arise in an uncontrolled fashion. In contrast to true major depression, however, these do not last long, and it is, in fact, the *instability* of the mood rather than the overall tone that is the abnormality. No one knows what causes this: ideas include damage to the commonly injured orbitofrontal parts of the brain (see, for example, Gurdjian et al., Journal of Trauma, 1976), chemical imbalances in the brain, and genetic predisposition brought out by the stress of brain injury (see Figure 10.1).

First priority: Assess Safety. Severe mood instability can lead to suicide. Admit the patient to a psychiatric ward if there are concerns about suicide or potential danger to others. Ask the patient and the collateral source directly, "Are you thinking about hurting yourself or anyone else?" and "Do you have a specific plan?" There is no evidence that asking these questions makes mood instability worse.

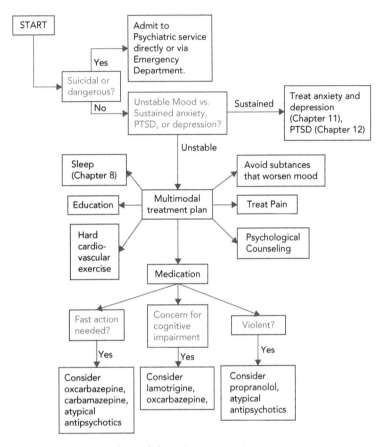

FIGURE 10.1 Mood instability after concussion.

Treatment

(1) First, determine whether the problem is actually mood instability, as opposed to generalized anxiety or major depression (Chapter 11), migraine aura manifesting as mood dysregulation (Chapter 7), or post-traumatic stress disorder (Chapter 12). These are best treated differently.

(2) Education

    a. Acknowledge that the problem is real, caused by the brain injury, and not the patient's fault.

    b. Give it a name: mood instability. Not depression, not "moral weakness," not selfishness.

    c. Help family members and others learn to redirect the patient, avoid inflammatory situations, and provide a calm and stable environment.

    d. Assure the patient and the family that it is an at least partially treatable condition.

    e. If the patient can afford it, some of this education can be best done by a professional psychologist with expertise in brain injury.

(3) Nonpharmacological interventions. *These are MORE important than the pharmacological strategies.*

    a. Improve sleep. Please see Chapter 8 for specific strategies to optimize sleep after concussion.

    b. Vigorous cardiovascular exercise:

        i. Consider writing an actual prescription: "30 to 60 minutes of hard cardiovascular exercise, 6 days per week *whether you feel like it or not, and an extra workout when your mood is unstable.*" Tell the patient and family to be as compliant with this prescription as they would be with a prescription for a medication or a referral to a surgeon.

        ii. Consider referral to physical therapy (PT) to help design an exercise program.

        iii. If the patient can afford it, 1 session per week with a personal trainer often can be very helpful to improve compliance.

    c. Treat migraine and other types of pain. All types of pain make mood instability worse. Please see Chapter 7 for specific strategies for the treatment of headache in the setting of concussion.

    d. Stop alcohol or other disinhibiting substances (but this is not the time to quit smoking or stop drinking coffee, because withdrawal from nicotine, THC, and caffeine can make mood instability worse).

    e. Stop offending medications: Levetiracetam (Keppra) for seizures is the most common mood-destabilizer.

    f. Cognitive-behavioral therapy optimally provided by a psychologist or therapist with experience with concussion patients. Cognitive-behavioral therapy can be very effective, but cost and finding the right provider are often issues.

(4) Pharmacological strategies, usually in addition to, not instead of the above nonpharmacological strategies. Several of these can be combined: often a cocktail of medications is best.

    a. Lamotrigine (Lamictal) may be the optimal mood stabilizer unless fast action is needed: It has the least cognitive side effects, it is generally weight neutral, it can be a "2 for 1" when there is a seizure disorder, and it is even relatively safe in pregnancy.

        i. Prescribe a starter pack, from 25 mg each day up to 100 bid over 2 months.

        ii. Standard dose is 100 mg bid but well tolerated at 200 bid or even higher.

        iii. Warn the patient and family about rash. It is extremely rare when the dose is increased slowly, but it can be a whole body, very severe rash if high doses are started right away. If there is a rash, stop the medication right away.

        iv. No drug level testing required, unless there is a question of whether the patient is actually taking the medication.

    b. Oxcarbazepine (Trileptal) is an excellent option when relatively fast action is needed. It is reasonable to prescribe oxcarbazepine for 2 months during the lamotrigine titration. It is safe to take both at the same time.

        i. Start at 300 mg bid, then increase to 600 mg bid in 1 week.

        ii. Monitor sodium levels: typically 1 week after each dose increase.

      iii. Can cause some somnolence, but typically well tolerated in young patients, better than carbamazepine (Tegretol).

      iv. No drug level testing required, unless there is a question of whether the patient is actually taking the medication.

  c. Carbamazepine (Tegretol): A good choice as a mood stabilizer when cost is an issue, but not quite as clean a side effect profile as lamotrigine or oxcarbazepine.

      i. Start 100 mg bid x 1 week, then 200 mg bid x 1 week, then 400 mg bid

      ii. Typical doses: 800 to 1600 mg total, divided into 2 to 3 doses per day

      iii. Monitor sodium levels: typically 1 week after each dose increase.

      iv. Monitor white blood cell counts and liver function: typically at least once a year.

      v. Drug-level testing can be helpful to assess whether side effects could be related to toxicity.

      vi. Complex drug–drug interactions. Worthwhile consulting with a pharmacist.

  d. Propranolol (Inderal)

      i. Can be a "2 for 1" as a migraine prophylactic as well.

      ii. A reasonable choice for reducing aggressive behavior after severe traumatic brain injury (TBI). Can be helpful after concussion as well. This is different than treatment of bipolar disorder.

      iii. Typical dosing: 20 mg tid x 1 week, then 40 mg tid x 1 week, then 60 mg tid. May need as high as 360 mg total daily dose.

      iv. Typically switch to long-acting formulation once the optimal dose is found.

      v. Dose-limiting side effects include orthostatic hypotension, bradycardia, reduced exercise tolerance, and less commonly, worsening depression.

vi. Relatively contraindicated in patients with asthma, hypotension, bradycardia, people performing or planning to perform hard cardiovascular exercise (which in itself is a good mood stabilizer), and poorly controlled depression.

e. Low dose of atypical antipsychotics, such as risperidone (Risperdal), quetiapine (Seroquel), and aripiprazole (Abilify)

   i. No clear preference for one over the other in terms of efficacy.

   ii. Aripiprazole (1 to 2 mg qhs) often chosen because it is associated with less weight gain than others.

   iii. Risperidone (0.5 to 1 mg bid) is the least expensive.

   iv. Quetiapine (5 to 10 mg bid) or rarely clozapine (Clozaril) are the best choices when parkinsonism is a comorbidity. Clozapine requires extensive monitoring of blood counts and is contraindicated when there is concern about irregular compliance with follow-up.

f. *Avoid* Valproic acid (Depakote). Valproic acid is *relatively contraindicated* because of cognitive side effects and weight gain. Worthwhile to switch to a different agent if the patient is already on it. Valproic acid is commonly prescribed by general psychiatrists without knowledge of concussion.

g. There is very little information or experience with lithium as a mood stabilizer in the setting of concussion. It requires extensive monitoring and is prescribed mainly by psychiatrists for true bipolar disorder.

h. In severe TBI, evidence is emerging that amantadine 100 mg po bid can be helpful to reduce agitation and aggression. No information about amantadine for this purpose after concussion yet.

i. There is ongoing interest in the use of dextromethorphan plus quinidine combination (Neudexta) as a mood stabilizer for traumatic brain injury patients. This combination is approved for pseudobulbar affect, a condition that involves expressions of emotion like laughing and crying without perception of the emotion itself. Little is known about its effects on mood instability in the setting of concussion, which is clearly different from pseudobulbar affect.

11

Anxiety and Depression

Anxiety and depression after concussion are quite treatable (see Figure 11.1).

First, assess safety. Severe anxiety and depression can lead to suicide. Once you have established that there is an issue with anxiety or depression and have established rapport, ask the patient and the collateral source directly about suicide. "Are you thinking about hurting yourself or anyone else?" "Do you have a specific plan?" There was some concern in the past that asking these questions might make the anxiety and depression worse, but this has not turned out to be the case. Admit the patient to a psychiatric ward if there are concerns about suicide or potential danger to others.

Second, distinguish between reactive anxiety and depressive symptoms vs. an impairing mood disorder. Reactive anxiety and depressive symptoms can be normal responses to a major change in life circumstances brought about by the injury and uncertainty about the future. Explain the difference between these two to the patient and the collateral source. A collateral source who knows the patient well before and after the concussion may have good insight.

If the patient has reactive anxiety and depressive symptoms but not an impairing mood disorder, the "treatment" is education, reassurance, and a good plan to get the patient's life back on track. Most patients want their life back the way it was before the injury. Often, they have been told that all their symptoms should have resolved and that they should be totally back to normal by now. It is true that between 70% and 95% of concussions do fully resolve quickly, but between 5% and 30% do not. Being part of this miserable minority

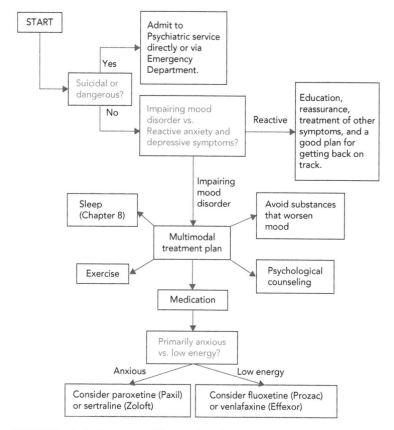

FIGURE 11.1 Anxiety and depression after concussion.

group without any explanation or clear way forward causes additional anxiety and depression. Often, education and getting started on a treatment plan for the most important symptoms relieves much of this sort of anxiety and depression.

If the patient has an impairing (but not immediately dangerous) mood disorder, start treating it right away as an outpatient. It should be treated for the most part just like a mood disorder in the absence of concussion, which can be done by nonpsychiatrists quite effectively for many patients.

The tools

(1) Exercise. Consider writing a prescription for exercise. This can be similar to the prescription used for attention deficit and mood instability described earlier; for example, "moderate cardiovascular exercise 30 minutes per day *whether you feel like it or not.*" Ideally, the patient should exercise with someone else to improve compliance and make it more enjoyable. Doing enjoyable activities is also part of cognitive behavioral therapy (see discussion later in this chapter).

(2) Treat sleep disturbances, usually with cognitive behavioral therapy for insomnia (Chapter 8). Cognitive behavioral therapy for insomnia has been shown to improve depression symptoms.

(3) Take a careful history of when anxiety symptoms occur relative to headaches. Sometimes, anxiety can be part of a migraine aura, coming minutes to hours before the headache phase (Gil-Gouveia et al., Journal of Neurology, 2015). Good treatment for migraine (Chapter 7) may reduce anxiety attacks if they are clearly correlated.

(4) Psychological counseling. Refer to a licensed therapist with expertise in treating mood disorders. The combination of therapy with medication is better than either alone. Specific options can include:

   a. Cognitive behavioral therapy designed to change the way the patients thinks about situations, correct misconceptions, and act more rationally. Refer to a psychologist or other therapist, ideally one with experience with concussion patients. The group at the University of Washington has adapted the principles of cognitive behavioral therapy for patients with impairments in information processing, attention, and memory. A recent randomized trial of cognitive behavioral therapy for depression in more severe traumatic brain injury (TBI) patients did not demonstrate effectiveness (Fann et al.,

Journal of Neurotrauma, 2015). In our experience, the benefits in concussion patients appear to be good.

b. Resilience training. A recent randomized controlled trial demonstrated reduced distress and anxiety after a 7-week course of resilience training designed for brain injury patients (Kreutzer et al., Brain Injury, 2018). The training was based on the concepts of cognitive behavioral therapy plus information from the book *Getting Better and Better after Brain Injury: A Guide for Survivors*.

c. Supportive psychotherapy designed to provide reassurance, encouragement, and comfort.

d. Interpersonal therapy designed to improve communication skills and focusing on interactions with other people.

e. Mindfulness-based therapy, involving focus on the immediate present. This includes meditation, training body awareness, and some yoga postures.

Not everyone has access to high-quality psychological counseling. Telephone-based cognitive behavioral therapy can be as effective as in-person therapy, though it may be delivered over a larger number of shorter sessions (e.g., 12 weekly sessions each 30 to 40 minutes long rather than 8 sessions each lasting a full hour).

(5) Avoid substances that worsen mood overall.

a. Avoid alcohol. In the first few weeks after concussion, no alcohol at all. In the longer-term, no more than 1 standard alcoholic drink in any 24-hour period. Although people feel a bit better in the short term, they do substantially worse in the long term.

b. Generally avoid marijuana. Although there are many claims that marijuana improves anxiety, in truth very little is known about this. There are also many examples of markedly impaired cognitive function due to marijuana. It isn't clear whether this is due to impurities or other drugs added to make it more addictive. It certainly causes weight gain, which can impair exercise tolerance. As marijuana becomes legal and more carefully regulated more will be learned about its role in concussion management.

c. Avoid short-acting benzodiazepines such as alprazolam (Xanax), diazepam (Valium), or lorazepam (Ativan) unless there is paralyzing anxiety. These medications impair cognitive function in the long term and have potential for misuse. Longer acting benzos like clonazepam aren't as bad, but they aren't the ideal choice either.

d. Avoid stimulants such as methylphenidate (Ritalin) in severe anxiety, but stimulants can be helpful in lethargic or melancholic depression.

e. Don't use high doses of propranolol. This and other central nervous system (CNS) acting beta blockers can worsen depression, though peripherally acting medications such as metoprolol (Lopressor, Toprol XL) are usually OK.

(6) Start an appropriate long-term antidepressant/antianxiety agent. There are many choices, but all take 4 to 6 weeks to be effective. All are only partially effective and by themselves they are not sufficient for optimal recovery.

a. Fluoxetine (Prozac) 10 to 20 mg each day. Increase up to 60 mg per day. Advantages: very potent antidepressant, improves energy, good long-term safety information. OK if the patient misses a dose (long half-life). Disadvantages: not very effective for anxiety, can worsen sexual performance.

b. Paroxetine (Paxil): 10 to 20 mg each evening. Increase up to 50 mg per day. Advantages: excellent for anxiety, good long-term safety information. Disadvantages: does not help energy levels, can worsen sexual performance.

c. Venlafaxine (Effexor) 37.5–75 mg extended release each morning, increase to 225 mg per day. Advantages: improves energy, fewer sexual performance side effects. Disadvantages: can slightly increase risk of seizures, can exacerbate migraine, not effective for anxiety.

d. Trazodone (Desyrel) 50 to 100 mg each evening. Increase up to 300 mg total daily dose. Advantages: improves sleep. Disadvantages: overall less effective antidepressant, causes some grogginess, lightheadedness, and "hangover."

e. Sertraline (Zoloft) 50 to 100 mg each evening. Increase up to 400 mg per day. Generally felt to be similar to paroxetine (Paxil). However, a randomized controlled study in traumatic brain injury patients within a year of injury found no benefit of sertraline versus placebo for depression (Fann et al., Journal of Head Trauma Rehabilitation, 2017). It is not clear whether this result is generalizable to other medications or other contexts.

f. Buspirone (Buspar): 10 mg po bid. Add-on therapy for anxiety. Not habit forming, low potential for abuse. Not much specific experience in concussion.

g. Mirtazapine (Remeron): reasonably effective in geriatric depression, improves sleep in lower doses. Not much specific experience in concussion.

h. Citalopram (Celexa) and escitalopram (Lexapro). Reasonably effective for depression and anxiety in other contexts. Not much specific experience in concussion.

i. Bupropion (Wellbutrin): Reasonably effective for depression and anxiety in other contexts. Improves smoking cessation. Not much specific experience in concussion. Relatively contraindicated in patients with seizure disorders.

Some concussion patients become very sensitive to the effects of small doses of antidepressants such that subfractionated doses are needed. A liquid formulation may be a good way to give someone 7.5 mg per day of paroxetine (Paxil) for example.

Importantly, offer the patient and collateral source a chance to follow up by phone, e-mail, or in person within 1 week after starting treatment for serious mood disorder. At the 1-week follow-up, assess for worsening mood disorder (especially suicidality) and adverse effects of medications. Then offer in-person follow-up in 6 to 8 weeks. If the patient is not doing better, re-evaluate using the same process. Consider further treatments for sleep, re-referral for psychological counseling, additional assessments for mood-impairing substances, increasing the dose of medication, and changing to a different medication.

Consider using a quantitative scale such as the Beck Depression Inventory, Patient Health Questionnaire 9 (PHQ9), or Beck Anxiety Inventory at each visit to assess the effects of treatment.

For patients with complex and refractory mood disorders, many effective options are available. Offer reassurance and refer to a psychiatrist promptly. It is a good idea to make the referral yourself rather than telling the patient to do so, given that patients with both concussion and a severe mood disorder may be less likely to follow through effectively.

Consider also managing the patient yourself in consultation with a psychiatrist. Some patients may accept treatment from a concussion clinic but may not be willing to go to see a psychiatrist because of concern about stigma. Effective options available in the concussion clinic include:

(1) Addition of mood stabilizers such as lamotrigine (Lamictal) or oxcarbazepine (Trileptal)
(2) Addition of stimulants such as methylphenidate (Ritalin)
(3) Addition of low doses of second-generation antipsychotics such as aripiprazole (Abilify), olanzapine (Zyprexa), quetiapine (Seroquel), or risperidone (Risperdal).

Consider referring the patient for *transcranial magnetic stimulation* treatment. Transcranial magnetic stimulation is approved by the U.S. Food and Drug Administration (FDA) for treatment of major depression. It can be a good choice for patients who don't want to or can't take medications. The therapy typically involves 20 daily outpatient sessions lasting less than 1 hour each. No anesthesia is involved. It is frequently covered by insurance if an adequate trial of an antidepressant medication has not been successful. The use of transcranial magnetic stimulation is rapidly expanding, and new methods for targeting the treatment are evolving quickly (Siddiqi et al., Journal of Neurotrauma 2018). The procedure is quite safe, with transient tension-type headaches being the most common side effect. The risk of seizures with transcranial magnetic stimulation is very low in general, and there is no evidence that concussion patients are at increased risk of seizures. Clearly, more severe TBI patients with penetrating injuries, temporal lobe hemorrhage, or hippocampal sclerosis are at higher risk for seizures and probably should not be treated with transcranial magnetic stimulation. Likewise, patients with metal implants or shrapnel should not be treated with transcranial magnetic stimulation; the contraindications are similar to those for magnetic resonance image (MRI) scanning.

12

Post-traumatic Stress Disorder

In many contexts, the trauma that caused the concussion can also trigger a strong stress response. A life-threatening car accident, a blast exposure from an industrial accident, assault, military combat-related injury, natural disaster, etc., can all increase the risk of post-traumatic stress disorder (PTSD). On the other hand, sports-related concussions, minor motor vehicle accidents, and simple falls usually do not increase the risk of PTSD. In the past, it was believed that loss of consciousness or amnesia would protect the patient from PTSD, but this is clearly not correct. In fact, it seems that concussive traumatic brain injury (TBI) increases the risk of PTSD, though why this occurs is not understood. PTSD treatment can be effectively started in the concussion clinic, and there is often less stigma associated with treatment in concussion clinic than in a psychiatric facility, so for some patients the concussion clinic is the best chance to diagnose and treat PTSD. It isn't productive to try to figure out exactly which problems are due to concussion and which are due to PTSD. It's impossible to do so with any reasonable degree of certainty, the combination is worse than each of them individually, and they are best treated together. The plan is as follows:

(1) Take a careful history.
   a. Ask specifically about feeling of horror, helplessness, dissociation, shock, or anguish during or immediately after the event that caused the concussion.
   b. Ask about current hyperarousal: sweating, shaking, and/or heart pounding in situations that remind the patient of the trauma.

c. Ask about nightmares: vivid dreams that wake the patient up and make it hard to get back to sleep. Sometimes patients are afraid to go to sleep.

d. Ask about avoidance: not going places or doing things that are related to the traumatic event.

e. Ask about emotional numbing: not feeling anything, not feeling normal closeness or affection toward family, friends, or previously enjoyed activities. *Although hyperarousal is the most classic symptom, emotional numbing is actually the most disabling.*

f. Ask about dissociation: a feeling of unreality, as though the patient isn't really there, and this isn't really happening.

g. Ask about prior PTSD. About 3% of the U.S. population has some level of PTSD at baseline, and it can be exacerbated by a concussive injury. Military personnel with partially compensated PTSD often deteriorate after a concussive injury.

h. CRITICAL: Ask the collateral source. Many patients don't want to talk about their PTSD symptoms because it makes the symptoms worse. Of course they don't want to talk about it; it's unpleasant and avoidance is one of the core symptoms.

(2) Assess safety. Severe PTSD can lead to suicide. Admit the patient to a psychiatric ward if there are concerns about suicide or potential danger to others. Ask the patient and the collateral source directly, "Are you thinking about hurting yourself or anyone else?" and "Do you have a specific plan?" It is safe to ask these questions. In the past, there was some concern that asking these questions might make the anxiety worse, but this has turned out not to be the case.

(3) Refer to a psychologist or counselor with specific expertise in PTSD, and ideally with expertise in concussion as well. This is the first-line treatment. The evidence is quite good that psychological treatment for PTSD is effective.

a. Prolonged Exposure Therapy. Requires 8 to 11 sessions plus homework exercises. There were initially some concerns that this therapy would not work in TBI patients because of their cognitive dysfunction, but recent evidence from the Veterans Administration (VA) system demonstrates reasonable effectiveness (Wolf et al., Journal of Traumatic Stress, 2015).

b. Cognitive Behavioral Therapy. Requires 8 to 11 sessions plus homework exercises.

c. New treatment methods are being tested. Consider referring the patient to a research center.

This can be expensive and not always covered by insurance, though it is provided by the VA system.

(4) Optimize sleep. See the section on sleep disorders after concussion (Chapter 8). This is a top priority for many patients with PTSD and *required* for optimal outcomes from prolonged exposure or cognitive behavioral therapy.

(5) Start an anxiolytic antidepressant. These take 4 to 6 weeks to be effective and should be considered as additions to optimization of sleep and prolonged exposure or cognitive behavioral therapy.

a. Paroxetine (Paxil) 10 to 20 mg po qhs, increasing up to 40 mg. Advantages: excellent for anxiety, good long-term safety information. Disadvantages: does not help energy levels, can worsen sexual performance.

b. Sertraline (Zoloft) 50 to 100 mg po qhs, increasing up to 200 mg. Similar to Paxil.

(6) Prescribe prazosin for nightmares. Start at 1 mg po qhs, then increase weekly by 1 mg until the nightmares improve or there are intolerable side effects. Most patients require 10 to 15 mg, but it can be tolerated up to 40 mg. There is double-blinded randomized controlled trial evidence for its effectiveness in some populations, especially those who are more severely affected (Raskind et al., The American Journal

of Psychiatry, 2013). If patients stop the medication, the nightmares can recur immediately. Common side effects include:

a. orthostatic hypotension

b. lethargy

c. dry mouth

(7) Ideally, use short-acting benzodiazepines such as alprazolam (Xanax), lorazepam (Ativan), and diazepam (Valium) only for emergencies. Some PTSD cases are so severe that the cognitive side effects may be worth it.

(8) Advise the patient to stop drinking alcohol. This is really hard to do, because many severe PTSD patients say that drinking is the only thing that lets them sleep. For overall health and cognitive recovery, however, it would be better to give the patient high doses of alprazolam (Xanax), lorazepam (Ativan), or diazepam (Valium) than have them drinking alcohol to excess every night—and they won't stop drinking unless they have something else to help them sleep. The benzodiazepines can be slowly tapered in a controlled fashion, whereas most people cannot slowly taper alcohol use.

Hierarchy: No sleep is the worst, alcohol-induced sleep is the second worst, benzodiazepine-induced sleep is the third worst, and natural sleep is the best.

(9) Treat chronic pain aggressively if present. All kinds of pain including migraines, musculoskeletal pain, and neuropathic pain worsen sleep and impair recovery from PTSD. Again, the cognitive side effects of narcotics, antiepileptics used for neuropathic pain, and migraine prophylactics are usually less impairing than the PTSD symptoms, so these side effects may be worth tolerating.

(10) Consider a second-line mood stabilizer if necessary. (Please also see Chapter 10.)

a. Lamotrigine (Lamictal) may be the optimal mood stabilizer unless fast action is needed. It has the least cognitive side effects, is generally weight neutral, can be a "2 for 1" when there is a seizure disorder, and is even relatively safe in pregnancy.

    i. Prescribe a starter pack, from 25 mg each day up to 100 bid over 2 months.

    ii. Standard dose is 100 mg bid but well tolerated at 200 bid or even higher.

    iii. Warn the patient and family about rash. It is extremely rare when the dose is increased slowly, but it can be a whole body, very severe rash if high doses started right away. If there is a rash, stop the medication immediately.

    iv. No drug level testing required, unless there is a question of whether the patient is actually taking the medication.

b. Oxcarbazepine (Trileptal) is an excellent option when relatively fast action needed. It is reasonable to prescribe oxcarbazepine for 2 months during the lamotrigine titration. It is safe to take both at the same time.

    i. Start at 300 mg bid, then increase to 600 mg bid in 1 week.

    ii. Monitor sodium levels: typically 1 week after each dose increase.

    iii. Can cause some somnolence, but typically well tolerated, better than carbamazepine (Tegretol).

    iv. No drug level testing required, unless there is a question of whether the patient is actually taking the medication.

c. Carbamazepine (Tegretol): A good choice as a mood stabilizer when cost is an issue, but not quite as clean a side effect profile as lamotrigine or oxcarbazepine.

    i. Start 100 mg bid x 1 week, then 200 mg bid x 1 week, then 400 mg bid

    ii. Typical doses: 800 to 1600 mg total, divided into 2 to 3 doses per day

    iii. Monitor sodium levels: typically 1 week after each dose increase.

      iv. Monitor white blood cell counts and liver function, typically at least once a year.

      v. Drug level testing can be helpful to assess whether side effects could be related to toxicity.

      vi. Complex drug–drug interactions; it may be worthwhile to consult with a pharmacist.

  d. Propranolol (Inderal)

      i. First choice for reducing aggressive behavior after severe TBI. Can be helpful after concussion as well. This is different than treatment of bipolar disorder.

      ii. Can be a "2 for 1" as a migraine prophylactic as well.

      iii. Typical dosing 20 mg tid x 1 week, then 40 mg tid x 1 week, then 60 mg tid. May need as high as 360 mg total daily dose.

      iv. Typically switch to long-acting formulation once the optimal dose is found.

      v. Dose-limiting side effects include orthostatic hypotension, bradycardia, reduced exercise tolerance, and less commonly, worsening depression.

      vi. Relatively contraindicated in patients with asthma, hypotension, bradycardia, people performing or planning to perform hard cardiovascular exercise (which in itself is a good mood stabilizer), and poorly controlled depression.

  e. Low dose of atypical antipsychotics; for example, risperidone (Risperdal), quetiapine (Seroquel), and aripiprazole (Abilify)

      i. No clear preference for one over the other in terms of efficacy.

      ii. Quetiapine (Seroquel) 25 mg bid up to 300 mg po qhs is commonly used in PTSD patients. It also helps with sleep because it is sedating. It may be the best choice when parkinsonism is a comorbidity. It causes weight gain, however, and can impair cognitive performance at high doses.

        iii. Aripiprazole (Abilify) 1 to 2 mg qhs is often chosen because it is associated with less weight gain than others.

        iv. Risperidone (Risperdal) 0.5 to 1 mg bid is the least expensive.

   f. Valproic acid (Depakote, Depakote ER) 500 to 1000 mg po total. Divided BID for regular, all qhs for the extended release.

        i. Relatively contraindicated after concussion due to sedation, cognitively impairing side effects, weight gain, and risk of birth defects.

        ii. Can be a benefit as a "2 for 1" migraine prophylactic or antiepileptic.

   g. Topiramate (Topamax) 25 mg po bid up to 150 mg po bid.

        i. Relatively contraindicated after concussion due to cognitive side effects ("dope-a-max")

        ii. If used, pay careful attention to hydration to reduce risk of kidney stones (very painful).

        iii. Can be a benefit to assist with weight loss and appetite suppression.

   h. Gabapentin (Neurontin) 300 mg po tid to 1200 mg po tid.

        i. Probably somewhat less effective than other agents.

        ii. Benefit may include improved pain control, especially in synergy with low-dose narcotics.

        iii. Few side effects or drug–drug interactions.

(11) Don't be afraid to use stimulants if the patient also has impairing attention deficit or there is another good reason to use them. In the past, it was believed that stimulants would worsen PTSD, but recent experience in military patients and others with both concussive TBI and PTSD has indicated that this does not occur *as long as the stimulant doesn't worsen sleep*. In fact, in a small randomized controlled trial of methylphenidate versus placebo, methylphenidate improved cognitive complaints and PTSD symptoms (McAllister et al., Neuropsychopharmacology, 2015). So,

modest doses of short-acting stimulants early in the day are not absolutely contraindicated. The situation is analogous to Tourette's syndrome, wherein it was believed that stimulants for commonly co-occurring ADHD would worsen tics, but this turned out to be incorrect. Caffeine may actually be more problematic than methylphenidate (Ritalin) for PTSD patients, given that it may be used in excess without the patient realizing it.

Consider using a quantitative scale such as the PTSD Checklist (PCL-5) at each visit to assess the effects of treatment.

The bottom line is that concussion care providers can (and often should) begin treating PTSD when it is apparent.

13

Personality Change

"Personality change" reported by the patient or collateral source can mean a lot of different things. Most common issues include mood instability, depression with loss of interests and pleasures, fatigue, loss of social intelligence, or other changes in interpersonal style such as reduced extraversion and conscientiousness. There can be more than one change at the same time.

The first question to consider is whether the personality change is an impairing problem as opposed to a nonimpairing (sometimes even beneficial) alteration.

If personality change is an impairing problem, treat any mood instability (Chapter 10), depression (Chapter 11), fatigue (Chapter 16), or loss of social intelligence. Treat pain aggressively (Chapters 7-8), because untreated pain makes most negative aspects of peoples' personalities worse, whether they've had a concussion or not.

For loss of social intelligence, make 2 referrals:

(1) To a trained psychologist with expertise in social intelligence assessment and treatment.
(2) To a speech or occupational therapist for rehabilitation of social pragmatics in a group setting. Given that social intelligence is so important for career success, this often falls under the expertise of a return-to-work program or occupational performance center. If the patient cannot afford an appropriate psychologist or one is not available, try to educate the patient and family by advising common-sense approaches. Strategies for impaired social intelligence include:

a. Making explicit the rules of social interaction so that they can be learned directly. This is similar to the approach used for high-functioning people on the autistic spectrum.

b. Modeling behavior using an actual or simulated peer group. The evidence in this field is pretty thin. In a recent randomized controlled trial, interactive group therapy was not shown to differ from the control intervention, which was group educational presentations. TBI patients in both groups improved modestly in social communication skills (Harrison-Felix et al., Archives of Physical and Rehabilitation Medicine, 2018). Furthermore, training to improve facial expression recognition did not improve empathy, irritability, or aggression (Neumann, Journal of Head Trauma Rehabilitation, 2015).

For other changes in interpersonal style that cause significant problems with work, family, or social life, consider referring the patient and family to a trained psychologist with expertise in personality disorders. There aren't any specific pharmacological treatments for interpersonal style.

If the personality change is not causing significant problems, it is usually sufficient to educate the patient and family:

(1) Personality commonly changes after brain injury.
(2) The changes do not seem to be a problem at the moment.
(3) Let us know if it gets worse or becomes a problem in the future.

14

Balance Problems

Balance is almost always acutely impaired after a concussion and recovers back to normal over 1 to 2 weeks. But when balance does not recover fully, this can be disabling for accomplished athletes and military personnel and substantially impairing for other individuals. Balance problems due to concussion can be especially troublesome if patients have comorbidities such as advanced age or peripheral neuropathy such that their balance was not so good at baseline. In fact, falling due to impaired balance may have been the reason the patient had a concussion in the first place. Address the following questions:

(1) "Is balance always a problem, or are there times when it is normal and then other times when it is really bad?" Episodic balance impairment is often quite treatable:
   a. Balance impairment due to intoxication by medications, alcohol, or other drugs can be treated by stopping the offending substance. Benzodiazepines used to treat anxiety or insomnia are common culprits. Use of a serotonin specific reuptake inhibitor (SSRI) and cognitive behavioral therapy can often make benzodiazepines unnecessary.
   b. An inner ear problem such as concussion-related benign paroxysmal positional vertigo can be treated with repositioning maneuvers. Perform the Dix-Hallpike maneuver in the office and look carefully at the patient's eyes for signs of nystagmus. The nystagmus is typically upbeat or rotational and may occur after a latency of up to 10 seconds. See video link http://www.youtube.com/watch?v=kEM9p4EX1jk and Figure 14.1). THIS IS CONTRAINDICATED IN PATIENTS WITH UNSTABLE

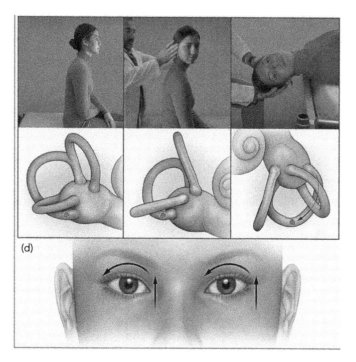

FIGURE 14.1 The Dix Hallpike Maneuver (right side). The maneuver should be repeated on the left side after resting 30 seconds. Reproduced with permission from Solomon, Current Treatment Options in Neurology, 2000.

NECK INJURY OR INSTABILITY. If it is positive, refer to physical therapy for repositioning maneuvers. Benign paroxysmal positional vertigo can actually be cured completely in some cases, which can be very gratifying for both the patient and the treating clinicians.

c. Migraine can cause intermittent balance problems. Even if there is no headache, migraine auras can impair balance. Treatment of migraine (Chapter 7) should be considered.

(2) "How much alcohol are you drinking these days?" Alcohol seems to impair the recovery of balance after concussion in

general, even when the patient is not actually drunk. Advise the patient to stop drinking, or at least cut down to a maximum of 1 alcoholic drink in any 24-hour period.

(3) If possible, have a physical therapist test balance.

a. In accomplished athletes and military personnel or other young healthy patients, consider using the BESS (balance error scoring system) from Riemann and Guskiewicz, Journal of Athletic Training, 2000. http://fs.ncaa.org/Docs/health_safety/BESS%20manual%20310.pdf

The BESS is not easy. Out of a possible 60 errors maximum, well-trained collegiate athletes without concussion make an average of 8 to 12 errors. Only special operations warriors and Olympians can complete the BESS. The foam pad tests are the most sensitive to concussion. Other scales, such as the Berg balance test, or simple tests like standing on 1 leg, are too easy for high-level athletes, and a normal performance does not reflect the actual impairment. If balance is impaired (more than 14 errors on the BESS, or abnormal performance compared to the patient's baseline), consider a referral to physical therapy specifically for balance training. A randomized (though unblinded) trial report indicated that an additional 8 weeks of specific balance training accelerated recovery of balance function and reduced dizziness compared to general rehabilitation in subacute traumatic brain injury (TBI) patients (Kleffelgaard et al., Clinical Rehabilitation, 2018).

b. In older patients or those with preexisting balance problems, use the Berg balance test. Again, refer to physical therapy specifically for balance training if abnormal.

(4) Consider prescribing additional self-directed balance exercises: tai chi, yoga, dance, practice walking on a low balance beam, etc. This takes a lot of time and effort for optimal results. Write out a prescription: "60 to 90 minutes of balance training, 3 to 6 days per week, *whether you feel like it or not.*"

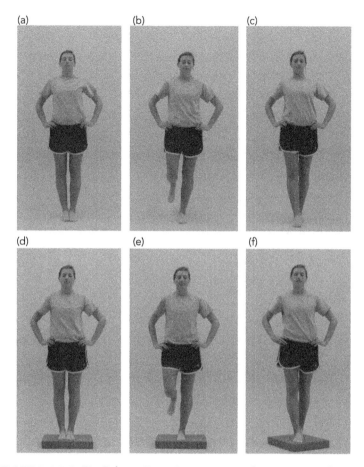

FIGURE 14.2 The Balance Error Scoring System has 6 parts, each 20 seconds long. Errors are counted if the patient lifts hands off the iliac crest, opens eyes, steps, stumbles, falls, moves hips into > 30- degree adduction, lifts foot or heel, or remains out of position for more than 5 seconds. Maximum 10 errors per position.

(5) Emphasize that balance training is also part of preventing future concussions. Often, after aggressive rehabilitation and training, the patient's balance may be *better* than it was before the concussion. Consider telling patients something like, "You are likely to recover well from this concussion, but

it will probably be harder to recover if you have another one. So, you need to do everything you can to prevent having another concussion, and balance training will help reduce the chance of a fall." (This is sometimes called "Vitamin S": the therapeutic scare).

15

Dizziness

Dizziness usually resolves rapidly, but if it does not, it can be a challenging chief complaint because it means so many different things to different people: lightheadedness, vertigo, poor balance, mental fogginess, and other concerns all can be called "dizziness" by the patient (see Figure 15.1).

First question: "When you say 'dizzy,' do you mean lightheaded like you might pass out, a spinning sensation like after a carnival ride, mental fogginess like you can't concentrate, or something else?"

IMPORTANT: The patient can have more than one of these at the same time, potentially indicating multiple problems that need to be addressed separately.

Perform a short screening test such as the VOMS (Vestibular Ocular Motor Screening).

This test involves asking whether symptoms worsen after testing smooth pursuit eye movements, saccadic eye movements, near point convergence, vestibular ocular reflex, and visual motion sensitivity. The best way to learn to perform the screening is by watching a video.

http://rethinkconcussions.upmc.com/2016/10/what-is-voms/
The detailed instructions can be found online:
https://www.physiotherapyalberta.ca/files/vomstool.pdf

Lightheadedness

Lightheadedness, meaning a feeling like the patient may pass out, is usually due to low blood pressure. Evaluate medications and check orthostatic blood pressures properly:

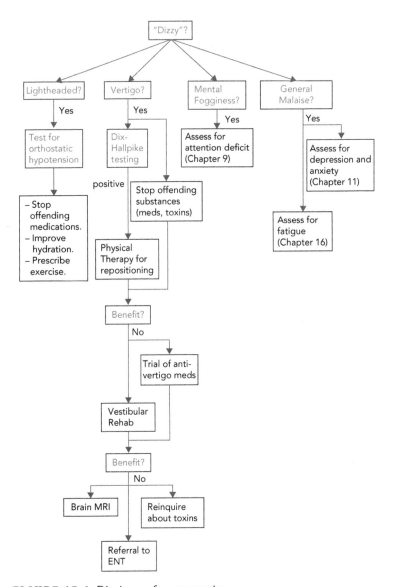

FIGURE 15.1 Dizziness after concussion.

(1) The patient should lie down for 5 minutes (you can obtain additional parts of the history in the meantime).
(2) Test blood pressure and heart rate.
(3) Have the patient sit up and ask the patient if this reproduces the dizziness.
(4) Check blood pressure and heart rate immediately. A drop in blood pressure and increase in heart rate indicate *transient orthostatic hypotension*.
(5) Wait 60 seconds and check blood pressure and heart rate again. A persistent drop in blood pressure and increase in heart rate indicate *persistent orthostatic hypotension*.
(6) Have the patient stand up and ask whether this reproduces the dizziness.
(7) Check blood pressure and heart rate immediately (transient orthostatic hypotension).
(8) Wait 60 seconds and check blood pressure and heart rate again (persistent orthostatic hypotension).

Transient orthostatic hypotension is usually due to central nervous system-acting medications or deconditioning. Taper and stop sedating medications such as benzodiazepines. Treat deconditioning with physical therapy and a prescription for regular exercise.

Persistent orthostatic hypotension can be due to blood pressure medications, dehydration, or autonomic instability. Educate the patient with regard to proper hydration and reduce beta blockers, calcium channel blockers, diuretics, etc. Although low blood pressure is a good long-term goal for cardiac and cerebrovascular health, the period of recovery from concussion is not the time to push the blood pressure too low. After concussion, some patients can become more susceptible to the side effects of medications they have been on chronically. Dehydration can be due to diuretic medications, headache with nausea and vomiting, poor oral intake due to depression or lethargy, impaired judgment leading to excessive exercise in hot weather, etc. Patients may need to liberalize salt in the diet as well as drink more water. In extreme cases, a brief urgent care clinic visit for 1 to 2 liters of normal saline (9 grams of salt per liter, a lot more than most people get in the diet) can make the patient feel a lot better.

If the lightheadedness doesn't respond to any of these measures, then consider autonomic instability. True autonomic instability is pretty rare after concussion. It is more common after severe traumatic brain injury (TBI) or spinal cord injury. Look for other additional factors such as diabetic peripheral neuropathy, toxic chemical exposure, rare neurological conditions related to Parkinson's disease (Parkinson-plus syndromes), or paraneoplastic syndromes related to several types of cancer. If you really think that the patient has autonomic insufficiency, this may require a referral to a neurologist who specializes in autonomic nervous system dysfunction for evaluation and treatment.

Vertigo

Vertigo, meaning a sensation of spinning or movement, can be an inner ear problem or a brain problem. First, follow Steps 1 through 3.

(1) Stop toxic substances. Narcotics, benzodiazepines, neuroleptics, older antiepileptics such as phenytoin (Dilantin) and phenobarbital, as well as many other medications can cause vertigo. Alcohol and many street drugs also can cause vertigo.

(2) Test lateral and up/down eye movements. If there is nystagmus, refer to ear, nose, and throat specialist (ENT) for a full evaluation.

(3) Perform the Dix Hallpike maneuvers in the office and look carefully at the patient's eyes for signs of nystagmus. The nystagmus is typically upbeat or rotational and may occur after a latency of up to 10 seconds (See video link http://www.youtube.com/watch?v=kEM9p4EX1jk and Figure 14.1). THIS IS CONTRAINDICATED IN PATIENTS WITH UNSTABLE NECK INJURY OR INSTABILITY. If these are positive, you can tell the patient that it is probably an

inner ear problem and that it is quite treatable. Send the patient to a specialized physical therapist for repositioning maneuvers. This can often fully resolve the problem.

If this doesn't fix the problem, then complete Step 4 and Step 5.

(4) Prescribe vestibular rehabilitation. A specialized physical therapist can teach the patient strategies to minimize the impact of vertigo in everyday life. There is evidence from randomized (though unblinded) trials that early cervical spine and vestibular physical therapy leads to faster return to sport participation in young athletes with persistent symptoms of dizziness, neck pain, and/or headaches. (Schneider et al., British Journal of Sports Medicine, 2014). In a more general TBI population, a randomized (though unblinded) trial report indicated that an additional 8 weeks of specific balance training accelerated recovery of balance function and reduced dizziness compared to general rehabilitation (Kleffelgaard et al., Clinical Rehabilitation, 2018). However, the control group caught up at later time points, so there was no net longer-term effect.

(5) Prescribe a scopolamine patch (Transderm Scop) for 1 week, plus additional dimenhydrinate (Dramamine) 50 to 100 mg or meclizine (Antivert) 12.5 to 25 mg as needed for situations likely to trigger vertigo. Don't use these longer unless absolutely necessary because of the anticholinergic effects on memory and attention. These medications may also delay the natural plasticity in the vestibular system. They help in the short term, but once the vestibular rehabilitation starts in earnest, they usually should be tapered or stopped.

If these still don't help, then complete Step 6, Step 7, and Step 8.

(6) Refer to a vestibular specialist, typically an ENT.

(7) Reinquire about toxic substances, heavy metal exposures, herbal or traditional remedies, narcotics or alcohol that perhaps the patient didn't tell you about the first time around. Ask the collateral source carefully.

(8) Order an magnetic resonance imaging (MRI) scan of the brain. Sometimes the concussion unmasks another unrelated problem, such as an acoustic neuroma, brainstem lesion, or cerebellar degeneration syndrome. If the scan is normal, this is reassuring. It doesn't tell you what is causing the vertigo, but it tells you that there aren't likely to be any big surprises.

Importantly, sometimes the cause of vertigo cannot be identified. There is still a lot we don't understand. Vertigo may gradually resolve on its own without specific treatment. Cognitive behavioral therapy can help coping skills for people who have to live with vertigo.

Mental Fogginess

Dizziness meaning "mental fogginess" usually turns out to be attention deficit (see Chapter 9).

Migraine

Migraine can cause intermittent dizziness. Even if there is no headache, migraine auras can impair balance. Treatment of migraine (Chapter 7) should be considered.

"Other" dizziness, meaning vague and nonspecific malaise, usually turns out to be fatigue, depression, or anxiety. See the sections on fatigue (Chapter 16) and depression and anxiety (Chapter 11).

16

Fatigue

It is quite common for patients to report that they are more fatigued chronically after a concussion: "I'm tired all the time now." "My energy level just never came back to normal."

A systematic approach to fatigue

(1) Figure out how bad it is. How much work, school, parenting, sports, recreation, socializing, and fun has the patient missed in the past month because he or she was too tired?

(2) Rule out the complaint of concussion-related fatigue as an excuse to get out of school, work, or unpleasant chores at home. Ask the collateral source about how fatigued the patient acts. "Does she miss out on fun or enjoyable things sometimes because she feels too tired?"

(3) Rule out depression. Depression causes profound loss of energy and can be at least partially treated with an activating antidepressant such as fluoxetine (Prozac) or venlafaxine (Effexor). But not all fatigued patients are depressed. Many are not, but they may become depressed later if the fatigue becomes chronic.

(4) Rule out a primary sleep disorder. If the patient is waking up 30 times per hour because of sleep apnea, of course he or she will be fatigued all the time. Virtually every patient with a complaint of significantly impairing fatigue should have a sleep study. Treatment of sleep apnea, restless leg syndrome, and unrecognized insomnia have a huge effect on fatigue. Cognitive behavioral therapy for insomnia has been shown to improve fatigue in traumatic brain injury (TBI)

patients (Nguyen et al., Archives of Physical Medicine and Rehabilitation, 2017).

(5) Rule out alcohol, sedating medications, and other drugs as a cause of fatigue. Common culprits include daytime benzodiazepines, antipsychotics, and some antiepileptics such as valproic acid (Depakote), phenytoin (Dilantin), and zonisamide (Zonegran). Typically, lamotrigine (Lamictal), levetiracetam (Keppra), or oxcarbazepine (Trileptal) cause the least fatigue. It's worth making a switch.

(6) Rule out withdrawal from stimulants. Stopping caffeine abruptly, for example, can cause substantial fatigue. Better to slowly taper caffeine. As a rule of thumb, decrease each week by no more than 1 regular small cup of coffee (100 mg caffeine) per day. Or maybe this isn't the time to stop drinking coffee.

(7) Rule out a systemic cause. Check blood pressure and oxygen saturation, then order a complete blood count (CBC), comprehensive metabolic panel (CMP), thyroid-stimulating hormone (TSH) test, and urinalysis. Hypotension, hypoxemia, renal failure, liver failure, anemia, hyponatremia, hypothyroidism, and chronic urinary tract infection are treatable causes of fatigue, whether they are related to concussion or not.

(8) Consider an endocrinological evaluation. Concussion rarely causes major endocrine dysfunction the way more severe TBI can, but if there are specific signs other than fatigue it may be worthwhile.

(9) Consider testing for vitamin D deficiency. An emerging literature suggests that 25-hydroxy vitamin D supplementation plus bright light exposure can improve fatigue in patients who are vitamin D deficient. Little is known about this in the setting of concussion.

(10) None of the above. Sometimes, the fatigue is purely caused by the concussion itself, or perhaps by other factors that have not yet been defined. This is an area where medical knowledge is not very advanced. In many cases, functional magnetic

resonance imaging (fMRI) scans indicate more widespread brain activation than typical, suggesting that perhaps the brain is doing more work to achieve the same results. In these cases, or if the reversible causes of fatigue have been reversed and the fatigue is still impairing, avoid blaming the patient and consider the following:

a. Prescribe a very gradually progressive exercise program: "5 minutes of light exercise each day for 1 week, then 7.5 minutes a day for 1 week, then 10 minutes, then 12.5 minutes, . . . until you get up to 30 minutes of light exercise per day, whether you feel like it or not." This is a standard treatment for chronic fatigue syndrome, but it is very different from cardiovascular exercise as a treatment for mood instability. Prescribing moderate or intense exercise not a good idea. It is likely to worsen fatigue: The patient will do it the first day, then be so overwhelmingly tired that he or she won't ever do it again.

b. Prescribe bright light treatment. Early morning exposure for 30 to 60 minutes to either the sun or a special lamp with lots of blue light (the kind used to treat seasonal affective disorder; e.g., Philips goLITE BLUE, Northern Light Technologies, or NatureBright). Initial randomized controlled trial evidence indicates that 4 weeks of daily blue light treatment reduced fatigue and daytime sleepiness following traumatic brain injury compared with yellow light treatment or no treatment (Sinclair et al., Neurorehabilitation and Neural Repair, 2014). The patient may need to keep using the light treatment indefinitely.

c. Stop all alcohol. Even 1 drink can significantly worsen fatigue.

d. For adults, consider a diet that is low in refined sugar. Anecdotally, this can improve fatigue in the long run. Sugar makes people more energetic for a few minutes, then more tired afterward.

e. In the most refractory cases, prescribe a stimulant such as methylphenidate (Ritalin) or amphetamine/dextroamphetamine (Adderall) with the same doses and same caveats as for attention deficit (Chapter 9). Often with the stimulant, the patient can begin to exercise every day. Consider making exercise compliance a condition of continuing to prescribe stimulants, because in the long term, regular exercise will be the most helpful.

f. Prescribe amantadine 100 mg q am, increasing to up to 400 mg per day. This antiviral medication has a modest effect on fatigue in multiple sclerosis patients, and anecdotally a similar benefit in concussion patients. It does not help attention deficit and is not as effective as true stimulants, such as methylphenidate (Ritalin) and amphetamine/dextroamphetamine (Adderall). But amantadine has fewer contraindications and side effects, so it's worth a try in patients who can't take stimulants.

g. Prescribe a trial of modafinil (Provigil) 100 mg po q am increasing to 200 mg po q am in 1 week. This wakefulness-promoting agent can be helpful, though again it is not as effective as a true stimulant for fatigue.

Consider using a quantitative measure such as The Fatigue Severity Scale on each visit to assess for benefits. This can sometimes be useful to demonstrate to patients that they are actually making progress even they are not aware of it.

http://geriatrictoolkit.missouri.edu/fatigue/Fatigue-Severity-Scale.pdf

17

Excessive Sleepiness

Many patients sleep a lot after concussion, especially in the first few days to weeks, but the definition of clinically important hypersomnia is excessive sleep that interferes with other aspects of life. Falling asleep too early, waking up too late, and falling asleep at the wrong time during the day are all included.

Take a careful history:

(1) What time do you fall asleep?
(2) What time do you wake up?
(3) What other times do you fall asleep during the day and for how long do you sleep?
(4) How much does excessive sleepiness interfere with your life?
(5) Ask the collateral source the same questions, in private if necessary.

Restrict driving if necessary. Anyone with a history of falling asleep while driving, regardless of whether they had an accident or not, should have driving privileges restricted until the cause of the hypersomnia can be determined and treated. Inform patient and the collateral source directly about driving restrictions. This is a difficult conversation, but an important one. A severely hypersomnolent patient can be just as dangerous as an epileptic patient, and laws just about everywhere restrict driving after a seizure.

If either the patient OR the collateral source indicates a significant impairment, then proceed to diagnosis and treatment:

(1) *Is the patient getting enough good-quality sleep at night?* Patient self-report often is not reliable. It is common for the patient

to say, "I sleep just fine at night," but then on a formal sleep study the patient can be found to have a severe (and often treatable) sleep disorder.

    a. Refer for an overnight polysomnogram ("sleep study") at a licensed sleep lab. Then treat any underlying disorders such as sleep apnea, restless leg syndrome, narcolepsy, or rapid eye movement (REM) sleep disorder.

    b. If the patient cannot get a polysomnogram right away, a sleep center may be able to arrange an at-home monitor. This provides some information about the worst offenders, such as sleep apnea.

    c. Ask the collateral source to watch the patient sleep for at least a few hours. Report back how many times the patient wakes up and goes back to sleep per hour and what caused the arousals (stopped breathing, restless legs, got up to go to the bathroom, no apparent reason, etc.).

(2) *Assess for depression.* Although insomnia is the classic symptom of Major Depressive Disorder, hypersomnia can also occur with various grades of depression after concussion. Specifically, inquire about low mood, hopelessness, helplessness, suicidal ideation, reduced interests and pleasures, etc. (See Chapter 11 for details). If appropriate, treat with an *activating* antidepressant:

    a. Fluoxetine (Prozac) 10 to 40 mg po q am

    b. Venlafaxine (Effexor) 75 to 225 mg po q am

    c. Switch from paroxetine (Paxil), sertraline (Zoloft), trazodone, mirtazapine (Remeron), or other relatively sedating antidepressants to an activating antidepressant. Make the switch gradually over 1 to 2 weeks, tapering the sedating antidepressant and ramping up the activating antidepressant.

    d. Consider switching from antidepressants that have variable effects on sleep from person to person, such as duloxetine (Cymbalta), citalopram (Celexa), or escitalopram (Lexapro).

(3) Take a careful medication history for *substances that can cause hypersomnia* and stop them if possible.

    a. Stop or reduce benzodiazepines: alprazolam (Xanax), lorazepam (Ativan), diazepam (Valium), clonazepam (Klonopin), etc.

    b. Stop or reduce neuroleptics such as quetiapine (Seroquel), risperidone (Risperdal), etc.

    c. Stop or reduce sedating antiepileptics such as valproic acid (Depakote), zonisamide (Zonegran), and phenytoin (Dilantin). If the patient needs an antiepileptic, switch to a less sedating choice such as Keppra or Lamictal.

    d. Stop or reduce anti-parkinsonism medications such as carbidopa-levodopa (Sinemet) and bromocriptine, which can cause "sleep attacks."

    e. Stop or reduce alcohol: Ask the collateral source in private.

    f. Stop or reduce illicit drugs, including marijuana. Even if it's legal, it's still a bad idea for people who sleep too much. Check a urine drug screen.

    g. Stop or reduce over-the-counter medications containing sedating antihistamines such as diphenhydramine (e.g., Benadryl and many others). These can make people sleepy in the daytime. Often the patient may not be aware that cold remedies and antiallergy medications can cause hypersomnia.

    h. Consider asking the patient to stop taking traditional or herbal remedies if very little is known about their effects in concussion.

    i. Inquire about recent withdrawal from caffeine or stimulants. Prescribe a taper over 2 to 4 weeks rather than an abrupt withdrawal.

(4) Rule out a systemic cause, as for fatigue (Chapter 16). Check blood pressure and oxygen saturation, then order a complete blood count, comprehensive metabolic panel, thyroid cascade, and urinalysis. Hypotension, hypoxemia, renal failure, liver failure, anemia, hyponatremia, hypothyroidism,

and chronic urinary tract infection can contribute to hypersomnolence.

(5) If the above specific factors have been evaluated and treated if appropriate, and the patient still has impairing hypersomnia, then move to additional treatment options. Mix and match. Many patients need more than one of these.

a. Prescribe a very gradually *progressive exercise* program: "5 minutes of light exercise each day for 1 week, then 7.5 minutes a day for 1 week, then 10 minutes, then 12.5 minutes, . . . until you get up to 30 minutes of light exercise per day, whether you feel like it or not." This is very different from the prescription for more intense exercise as a mood stabilizer.

b. Prescribe a trial of *caffeine*: 100 mg first thing in the morning and 100 mg after lunch. Increase by 50 to 100 mg each week until there is a benefit or side effects. *Contraindications to caffeine include poorly controlled hypertension, tachycardia, severe anxiety, and certain cardiac arrhythmias.* Dose-limiting side effects include hypertension, tachycardia, anxiety, insomnia, and headache. For reference:

   i. Regular coffee: 95 to 200 mg per 8 oz cup
   ii. Espresso coffee: 40 to 75 mg per 1 oz shot
   iii. Typical soft drinks: 30 to 50 mg per 12 oz can
   iv. Tea: 15 to 60 mg per 8 oz cup
   v. Energy drinks (e.g., Red Bull, Rockstar, or Monster): 50 to 200 mg per can
   vi. Caffeine-containing headache medications (e.g., Excedrin Migraine): 65 mg
   vii. Over-the-counter caffeine tablets (e.g., NoDoz): 200 mg per tablet.

To avoid tolerance, recommend caffeine use 6 days per week rather than 7 and 51 weeks per year rather than 52.

c. Prescribe a trial of *modafinil* (Provigil) or armodafinil (Nuvigil). Modafinil is dosed at 100 mg po q am, then if necessary, increasing by 100 mg po each week to a maximum dose of 400 mg per day. Armodafinil is dosed at 150 to 250 mg per day. Armodafinil is longer acting. These wakefulness promoting agents (not stimulants) can be helpful for idiopathic hypersomnia. Unlike caffeine and stimulants, they do not typically cause tolerance or increase heart rate. However, getting insurance companies to pay for them can be challenging. Even generic versions can cost hundreds of dollars per month.

d. In the most refractory cases, prescribe a *stimulant* such as methylphenidate (Ritalin) or amphetamine/dextroamphetamine (Adderall), with the same doses and same caveats as for attention deficit (see Chapter 9). Stimulants can be used in combination with modafinil and caffeine. Small doses of each may be better tolerated than a large dose of a single agent.

e. Give basic advice regarding daily planning; for example, schedule the most important activities for times when the patient is most likely to be fully awake, such as mid-morning.

Administer the Epworth sleepiness scale to quantitatively track progress: http://yoursleep.aasmnet.org/pdf/Epworth.pdf

18

Memory Impairment

Upon taking a careful history, many complaints of memory problems actually turn out to be attention deficit (see Chapter 9). True memory loss is pretty rare after concussion. A complaint about "short term" memory: "I forget where I left my keys," "I can't remember people's names that I just met," etc., often is due to attention deficit. True memory problems are indicated by complaints such as, "I said his name 5 times to myself after I met him, and I still couldn't remember it the next day." Or, "He's getting lost in our own neighborhood."

It is important to distinguish them, because attention and memory are optimally treated differently. If both memory and attention are significant concerns, both should be treated (see Chapter 9).

It is also important to ask about the *emotional context*. Patients with mood instability can get overwhelmed by emotionally charged situations and have poor memory performance as a result. If this appears to be the case, treat the mood instability first.

In the clinic, consider performing simple tests of 3 types of memory:

(1) Verbal: repeat back 3 unrelated words immediately, then recall them at 5 minutes. Normal performance is correct recall of at least 2 of the 3 words and the third word recalled after a hint.

(2) Visuospatial: hide 3 colored pens around the exam room and ask the patient to find them 5 minutes later. Normal performance is all 3 found. Important not to give verbal cues to the patient.

TABLE 18.1 How Do You Tell the Difference between Problems with Memory versus Attention?

	Memory Impairment	*Attention Deficit*
Formal Neuropsychological Testing	Impairment on quantitative and standardized tests of immediate and delayed recall.	Impairment on quantitative and standardized tests of sustained vigilance, reaction times, and working memory.
Bedside Cognitive Testing	Errors on informal tests of immediate and delayed recall.	Errors on informal tests of sustained attention to task.
Everyday Life Symptoms	Getting lost. Losing things permanently and not being aware of the loss. Forgetting important people, places, and events. Difficulty learning new facts or new skills.	Misplacing things but finding them again later. Trouble staying focused on tasks. Trouble restarting a task after an interruption.
Source	Patient may or may not be aware of the deficits. Often more troubling to others than to the patient.	Concerning to both patient and others.

(3) Motor learning: show the patient the Luria sequence, let him practice it with each hand until it is done correctly, then ask him to do it again 5 minutes later. For the Luria sequence, tap a table with the fist, the side of the hand, and then the palm. Important not to give verbal cues. Normal

performance is learning the sequence within the second try, then recalling it correctly with no errors.

These tests are fairly easy for high-functioning people even after concussion, and a perfect performance does not mean that memory is not impaired.

Consider alternatively performing a standardized short quantitative test such as the Montreal Cognitive Assessment (MoCA) http://www.memorylosstest.com/dl/moca-test-english-7-1.pdf

Neuropsychological testing

If the history is not clear or if medico-legal documentation is required, order formal neuropsychological testing. This testing can be expensive, and it is not always covered by insurance. It can, however, clearly distinguish between memory loss and attention deficit (or document the presence of both), assess the severity quantitatively to track improvement or deterioration over time, and to some extent guide strategies for rehabilitation.

Caveats: There are 3 major limitations of neuropsychological testing:

(1) It is expensive, not always covered by insurance, and not always available in a timely manner.
(2) It does not compare the patient to his or her own preinjury baseline. A patient who may have been 90th percentile before injury and is functioning at 40th percentile after injury will be scored as "normal" even though he or she is clearly impaired in the real world compared to baseline.
(3) The testing is performed in a quiet, nondistracting setting and the tests do not have much emotional salience. Real world performance in distracting environments or involving emotionally charged tasks may differ substantially.

Thus, just like a radiological study, the rule is "treat the patient, not the test result." If the patient and collateral sources clearly indicate memory problems in the real world and the neuropsychological test results indicate normal memory, still treat the patient for memory problems.

Treatment

Each of these approaches alone has a small effect. For optimal treatment, use ALL of them.

(1) Reduce or eliminate barriers to optimal memory function.
   a. *Optimize sleep* (see Chapter 8). Sleep should be not just adequate but optimal. The patient should be fully refreshed. It may take months for the adverse effects of chronic sleep deprivation on memory to resolve. Optimal sleep is recommended as a strategy that might delay the onset of age-related cognitive impairment as well.
   b. *Treat chronic pain.* Ideally, treat with non-narcotic medications and nonpharmacological strategies. However, untreated severe pain impairs memory more than narcotics. Narcotics actually improve memory in patients with severe, untreated chronic pain if they allow the patient to sleep at night and concentrate during the day. This is often an issue in athletes with multiple orthopedic injuries, military personnel, and other poly-trauma patients.
   c. Take a careful history of when memory problems occur relative to headaches. Sometimes, memory problems can be part of a migraine aura, coming minutes to hours before the headache phase (Gil-Gouveia et al., Journal of Neurology, 2018). Good treatment for migraine (Chapter 7) may reduce memory problems if they are clearly correlated in time.
   d. Taper and stop cognitively impairing medications as much as possible.

      i. *Avoid* benzodiazepines such as alprazolam (Xanax), lorazepam (Ativan), diazepam (Valium), and clonazepam (Klonopin).

     ii. *Avoid* antipsychotics such as risperidone (Risperdal), quetiapine (Seroquel), aripiprazole (Abilify), and haloperidol (Haldol).

    iii. *Avoid* sedating antiepileptics such as valproic acid (Depakote), phenytoin (Dilantin), zonisamide (Zonegran), and possibly lacosamide (Vimpat, though little is known about the effects of Vimpat in concussion patients).

    iv. *Avoid* anticholinergics such as diphenhydramine (Benadryl), scopolamine patch (Transderm Scop), dimenhydrinate, (Dramamine), and meclizine (Antivert). Unmedicated sleep is best, so cognitive behavioral therapy for insomnia is the best choice, but zolpidem (Ambien) and eszopiclone (Lunesta) have less effect on memory than anticholinergic agents.

e. *Stop alcohol.* Unrecognized alcohol abuse can be the primary cause of memory loss. Often the full extent of alcohol use will not be apparent on the first visit. It takes time and trust. If it is apparent that alcohol is the problem, give advice to stop in a sensitive and nonjudgmental way. Make appropriate confidential referrals to rehab if the patient is willing.

f. *Stop other illicit drugs.* Many drugs, including marijuana, can substantially impair memory performance. Again, this may not be apparent on the first visit. A careful collateral history taken in private or by phone on another day may be the best way to sort this out. If it is apparent that drugs are the problem, give advice to stop in a sensitive and nonjudgmental way. Make appropriate confidential referrals to rehab if the patient is willing.

g. Moderate cardiovascular *exercise* helps memory performance. Consider writing a prescription for "30 to 60 minutes of moderately intense cardiovascular exercise 6 days per week whether you feel like it or not."

h. Test for vitamin B12 deficiency, hypothyroidism, electrolyte disorders, hypo- or hyperglycemia, renal failure, liver failure, and anemia. Treat abnormalities if present. It is not common for these to be the main cause of new-onset memory impairments after concussion.

i. This may not be the time to stop smoking, given that nicotine improves memory function. On the other hand, a nicotine patch can be just as effective as smoking without the other health risks.

(2) *Cognitive rehabilitation*: Refer to speech therapy and occupational therapy for memory training. This training can involve:

a. Learning compensatory strategies
   i. Regular calendar use with reminders
   ii. Notetaking
   iii. "To do" lists
   iv. Using smart phones or other assistive electronic devices
   v. Systematics (e.g., putting things in the same place every time)

This can be individual or group based. In a randomized, controlled (though not fully blinded) trial of a 12-week manual-based educational and compensatory approach called CogSMART, the authors reported improved memory for real world tasks 24 hours after being reminded, as well as improved overall symptoms and quality of life 1 year later (Twamley et al., Journal of Head Trauma Rehabilitation, 2015). In another randomized (though not fully blinded) trial of 10 weeks of group-based compensatory cognitive training, the authors reported improved self-reported cognitive and memory difficulties, greater use of cognitive strategies, and improvements on neurocognitive tests (Storzbach et al., Journal of Head Trauma Rehabilitation, 2017). Importantly, the benefits were similar for traumatic brain injury (TBI) patients with post-traumatic stress disorder (PTSD) and depression as well, though the benefits in those with substance abuse was not fully assessed (Pagulayan et al., Archives of Physical Medicine and Rehabilitation, 2017).

b. Memory-enhancement strategies
   i. Spaced rehearsal: repeat or paraphrase immediately, again at 5 minutes, again at 30 minutes, again the next day. (This is commonly used in foreign language training.)
   ii. Method of loci: associating the items to remember with a very familiar place, then mental rehearsal of moving through the place (the ancient Greeks used this to memorize long poems). This may be hard for some concussion patients.
   iii. Chunking: grouping numbers or elements into larger bits: It is easier to remember two 3-digit numbers and two 2-digit numbers than 10 individual digits in a telephone number.
   iv. Emotionally salient associations. Making up a funny, sad, or exciting story involving the items to be remembered triggers stronger associations than emotionally neutral memorization. Medical students use this approach a lot.
   v. Adaptive working memory training using computer-based systems. A small randomized controlled trial of an adaptive working memory training system (Cogmed) in children with moderate-to-severe TBI demonstrated improvement in reading comprehension and accuracy (Phillips et al., Journal of Neurotrauma, 2016). However, the effects in concussion patients and in other demographic groups have not been reported.
   vi. Cognitive rehabilitation using an intervention called Memory and Attention Adaptation Training combined with methylphenidate can be more beneficial

for nonverbal learning than either therapy alone (McDonald et al., Neuropsychopharmacology, 2017).

(3) Pharmacological enhancers of memory (nootropic agents). More than one can be used together.

a. *Caffeine:* 1 to 2 cups of coffee per day or the equivalent no later than 8 hours before bedtime can substantially enhance memory in caffeine-naïve patients. Risks include worsening headache, worsening anxiety, tachycardia, and worsening hypertension. Use caffeine 6 days per week, 51 weeks per year to prevent tolerance from developing.

b. *Donepezil* (Aricept): 5 mg po qd x 14 days, then 10 mg po qd. There is no clear additional benefit of the higher 23 mg dose in concussion patients. This acetylcholinesterase inhibitor increases acetylcholine at the synapses, having the opposite effect of anticholinergic medications. It is FDA-approved for Alzheimer's disease and Dementia with Lewy Bodies, but has a modestly beneficial effect after TBI and improves memory performance a little bit in normal subjects as well.

    i. Side effects: most commonly gastrointestinal (GI) upset, nausea, and diarrhea. These typically resolve within 2 weeks after each dose increase.

    ii. Risks:

        1. Worsening headaches. If intolerable, this may limit use.

        2. Worsening seizure disorder. Not common, but relatively contraindicated in uncontrolled seizures.

    iii. Duration of therapy: no long-term adverse effects in treatment for many years.

c. *Rivastigmine* (Exelon): 1.5 mg po bid x 14 days, then 3 mg po bid x 14 days, then 6 mg po bid. Similar to donepezil.

d. *Rivastigmine* transdermal (Exelon patch): 4.6 mg per day, or 9.5 mg per day. May have fewer GI side effects. Worth a try if donepezil is beneficial but the GI side effects are troubling.

e. *Stimulants*: beneficial for attention deficit and fatigue. Importantly, stimulants may allow the patient to do more intense cognitive rehabilitation, especially if cognitive rehabilitation is limited by fatigue. Consider regular short-acting methylphenidate (Ritalin) 5 to 10 mg 30 min before each intensive cognitive rehabilitation session. See Chapter 9 for detailed information on contraindications and appropriate monitoring.

f. *Modafinil* (Provigil): 100 to 200 mg each morning or armodafinil (Nuvigil) 150 to 250 mg each morning. No direct effect on memory, but there may be benefit if cognitive rehabilitation is limited by sleepiness.

g. Memantine (Namenda), amantadine, D-cycloserine, vitamins, ginkgo-biloba, taurine, ginseng, and other supposed nootropic agents: unknown whether there is benefit in concussion. A randomized controlled trial of amantadine demonstrated that there was no benefit in chronic TBI patients with a mixture of injury severities (Hammond et al., Journal of Neurotrauma, 2018).

h. Possible role for glucose in children and adolescents; for example, 100 to 200 calories of a high glycemic index snack or drink just before tasks requiring memory may improve performance. Not as clear in adults.

Note that it is important to use the short-acting pharmacological methods *in coordination* with cognitive rehabilitation; that is, methylphenidate (Ritalin) or caffeine 30 minutes before each cognitive training session, glucose right before the session.

These approaches can also improve memory in people who have not had a concussion, or whose concussion symptoms have resolved. With these strategies, memory may end up better than it was prior to concussion. The concussion symptoms may resolve, and the patient may continue to use the strategies and medications in everyday life. This can sometimes blur the line between treatment and augmentation.

19

Executive Dysfunction

Problems with organization, planning, strategy decisions, mental flexibility, optimizing risk/reward relationships, prioritizing, and goal setting are often lumped together and called executive dysfunction. These problems are common after more severe traumatic brain injury (TBI), but less common after concussion. As with memory impairments (Chapter 18), many of the failures in these domains are actually due to attention deficit or mood instability. There are no really good office-based tests of executive function. Just as with memory impairments, collateral history and neuropsychological testing (with the same caveats) will help sort out the nature of the impairment. Remember, the rule is "treat the patient, not the test result."

Treatment

(1) As with memory impairments, reduce or eliminate barriers to optimal executive function.
   a. Optimize sleep.
   b. Treat chronic pain, ideally with non-narcotic medications and nonpharmacological strategies.
   c. Taper and stop cognitively impairing medications as much as possible.
      i. Benzodiazepines
      ii. Antipsychotics
      iii. Sedating antiepileptics
      iv. Anticholinergics such as diphenhydramine (Benadryl), scopolamine (Transderm Scop), dimenhydrinate (Dramamine), or meclizine (Antivert).

    d. Stop or minimize alcohol.

    e. Stop other illicit drugs, including marijuana.

    f. Moderate cardiovascular exercise may help executive function, but it is not as clear as for memory in the setting of TBI. The benefits of exercise are better documented for early Alzheimer's disease. Specific regimen:

      i. 4 days per week for 6 months to achieve a benefit.

      ii. 15 minutes of warm-up followed by 30 to 45 minutes per day of moderate to intense cardiovascular exercise (at least 70% of maximum heart rate).

      iii. 1-on-1 personal trainer/coach to improve compliance and prevent injury. This is expensive but often helpful.

(2) Cognitive rehabilitation: Refer to speech therapy and occupational therapy for executive function training. This training can involve

    a. Dividing complex tasks into manageable bite-sized pieces, then executing them one at a time.

    b. Practice talking through potential decisions with trusted advisors before making them.

    c. Practice making organizational flow charts.

    d. Effectively using calendars, reminders, and other electronic organizational tools.

    e. Practicing strategic "if-then" flow charts.

    f. Making lists and then reordering them according to priority.

    g. Listing pros and cons of potential decisions.

(3) Pharmacological enhancers of overall cognitive function: There aren't really any specific agents for executive dysfunction.

    a. Caffeine if fatigue or sleepiness are limiting

    b. Stimulants if fatigue, initiation, or attention are limiting

    c. Donepezil (Aricept) or rivastigmine (Exelon) if memory is limiting

    d. Modafinil (Provigil) if sleepiness is limiting

e. Perhaps a role for dopaminergic agonists such a bromocriptine, but this has not been well established.
f. Possible role for glucose; for example, 100 to 200 calories of a high glycemic index snack or drink, to improve performance *especially in children and adolescents*. Not as clear in adults.

20

Parkinsonism

The classic triad of parkinsonism from all causes (not just Parkinson's disease) includes

(1) Bradykinesia: slowness of movement and speech.
(2) Rigidity: increased resistance of the arms, legs, neck, and torso to passive movement.
(3) Tremor: typically in the hands or arms; present at rest, but not with movement.

Balance impairment is also a major problem.

Parkinsonism can be a delayed consequence of multiple concussions. Parkinsonism is often, but not always part of chronic traumatic encephalopathy (see Chapter 36). There is an increased risk of parkinsonism after a single concussion, but the increased risk is modest and it's not always clear which comes first—undiagnosed parkinsonism causing a fall or other accident, or the injury causing the parkinsonism. The order of causality usually doesn't matter except in a medico-legal context. Treat the patient.

Parkinsonism is usually due to damage to the dopamine containing neurons in the midbrain or the axons from these neurons running to the striatum. At present, there is no accurate way to tell how much injury there is to these systems in living patients. A normal scan does not rule out damage to the dopamine system. Treat the patient, not the scan results (see Figure 20.1).

First, examine the patient:

(1) Assess for bradykinesia.
   a. Watch the patient walk, turn, and pass through a doorway. Parkinsonian patients may shuffle, have reduced arm

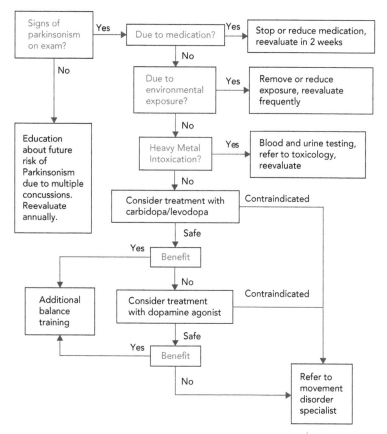

FIGURE 20.1 Parkinsonism after multiple concussions.

    swing, take short steps, require many steps to turn, and get stuck in a doorway.

    b. Have the patient pretend to "screw in a light bulb" with each hand. Slow and irregular movements are a hallmark of parkinsonism.

    c. Watch the patient's face at rest. Reduced facial movement and reduced blink rate are classic findings.

(2) Assess for rigidity.

    a. Have the patient relax as much as possible, then move the patient's wrist, arm, and shoulder slowly, then more quickly. Test both sides. Then do the same for both legs. Rigidity is increased resistance to motion that is similar when the examiner moves slowly or moves quickly. Spasticity (which is not a part of parkinsonism), in contrast, involves increased resistance when the examiner moves quickly.

    b. Gently move the patient's neck (if there are no injuries) to assess for rigidity in the neck.

(3) Assess for tremor.

    a. Have the patient place both hands on his or her lap and watch them at rest. Parkinsonian tremor is slow and worse at rest.

    b. Have the patient open and close one hand. The tremor in the other hand may worsen in parkinsonism.

    c. Have the patient extend both hands. Parkinsonian tremor decreases with posture, but other kinds of tremor may increase, such as essential tremor and tremor caused by stimulants.

    d. Have the patient touch your finger, his or her nose, then your finger back and forth as fast as possible. Parkinsonian tremor decreases with action, but other kinds of tremor such as that due to cerebellar injury may worsen.

(4) Test balance. See Chapter 14.

If the patient has parkinsonism, *the first priority is to determine whether there is a reversible cause, most commonly a medication.*

(1) Nearly all antipsychotic/neuroleptic medications and some antinausea medications can cause a drug-related parkinsonism because they block dopamine receptors. The effects of medications can be fully reversible once the medication is stopped. Common offenders include:

    a. Risperidone (Risperdal) or haloperidol (Haldol) for agitation. Stop this, address the underlying cause of agitation and substitute another medication such as propranolol (Inderal), lamotrigine (Lamictal), or oxcarbazepine (Trileptal), if appropriate (see Chapter 10).

b. All but a few neuroleptics for psychosis worsen parkinsonism. In consultation with a psychiatrist, gradually transition off of the other antipsychotic and onto quetiapine (Seroquel), olanzapine (Zyprexa), or clozapine (Clozaril), which generally do not cause parkinsonism. Avoid an abrupt switch, to reduce the risk of breakthrough psychosis.

c. Prochlorperazine (Compazine), metoclopramide (Reglan), or promethazine (Phenergan) for nausea. Substitute ondansetron (Zofran) or dronabinol (Marinol), though Marinol can cause psychosis with chronic use.

d. Some antidepressants such as citalopram (Celexa), escitalopram (Lexapro), bupropion (Wellbutrin), and fluoxetine (Prozac) have been associated with worsening parkinsonism. Consider switching to paroxetine (Paxil), mirtazapine (Remeron), venlafaxine (Effexor), or sertraline (Zoloft).

It may take 2 weeks or more for the effects of these medications to wash out. Fluoxetine has an especially long half-life. If there are still signs and symptoms of parkinsonism after 2 weeks off of all offending medications, there may be an underlying injury that was unmarked by the medication and needs to be treated separately.

(2) Assess for heavy metal intoxication with blood and urine tests. Manganese intoxication is rare, but it can cause parkinsonism and can be treated with ethylene diamine tetraacetic acid (EDTA) chelation therapy. Refer to a toxicologist with expertise in this topic.

(3) Inquire about exposure to environmental hazards such as manganese mining, welding, and pipefitting. Stop exposure. Recommend switching jobs if possible. The parkinsonism may be partially reversible, and most importantly, is less likely to continue to progress once the exposure is removed.

Pharmacological Treatment

If the patient has parkinsonism, and it is not due to one of the reversible causes above, consider pharmacological treatment. The goal is to reduce signs and symptoms to a tolerable level, not to eliminate them completely.

(1) Carbidopa–levodopa combination (Sinemet).
   a. Start with a half tablet of the 25 mg/100 mg combination 3 times per day.
   b. Increase by half tablet tid every 2 weeks until signs and symptoms are tolerable, or side effects occur. Side effects include
      i. Nausea. Usually resolves after 1 to 2 weeks of a dose increase. Don't use prochlorperazine (Compazine), metoclopramide (Reglan), or promethazine (Phenergan). Substitute ondansetron (Zofran) or dronabinol (Marinol), though Marinol can cause psychosis with chronic use.
      ii. Hallucinations. Usually visual. Consider dose reduction or addition of quetiapine (Seroquel), olanzapine (Zyprexa), or clozapine (Clozaril).
      iii. Orthostatic hypotension. Consider reducing blood pressure medications, liberalizing salt in the diet, optimizing hydration, and using compression stockings.
      iv. Sleep attacks. Consider restricting driving, using modafinil (Provigil), or reducing dose.
      v. Dyskinesias. These involuntary writhing movements usually occur after many years of treatment and typically require dose reduction. Refer to a movement disorders specialist for advanced options.
      vi. Dystonias. These involuntary postures, such as neck twisting, can present right away, or years later. They

usually require dose reduction. Refer to a movement disorders specialist for advanced options.

c. Doses higher than 12 tablets of carbidopa–levodopa (Sinemet) per day are rarely beneficial. This medication acts by supplementing dopamine in the nerve terminals. It only works if there are nerve terminals present and does not work if they have been destroyed. If it is not effective, stop it and switch to a dopamine agonist (see discussion later in this chapter).

(2) Bromocriptine (Parlodel): a dopamine agonist that acts directly on the receptors and may work even if carbidopa–levodopa (Sinemet) does not.

a. Dose: 5 mg po bid, increasing by 5 mg bid every 2 weeks until the parkinsonian signs and symptoms are tolerable, or side effects occur. Doses greater than 30 mg bid are rarely effective.

b. Side effects:

i. Confusion or hallucinations. Requires dose reduction.

ii. Orthostatic hypotension. Consider reducing blood pressure medications, liberalizing salt in the diet, optimizing hydration, using compression stockings, or reducing dose.

(3) Other dopamine agonists, such as ropinirole (Requip), pramipexole (Mirapex), rotigotine (Neupro patch), and apomorphine (Apokyn injection). Commonly used in Parkinson's disease but little experience in concussion-related parkinsonism patients.

(4) *Avoid anticholinergics* used for Parkinson's disease, such as benztropine (Cogentin), biperiden (Diovan), procyclidine (Kemadrin), and trihexyphenidyl (Artane), which may worsen cognitive function in concussion patients.

Safety: Importantly, parkinsonism increases the risk for falls, which can then cause further injuries. In addition to optimizing pharmacological treatment, also refer to physical therapy for balance training and education on how to reduce fall risk.

Prognosis: Importantly, multiple concussion-related parkinsonism is not the same as Parkinson's disease. Injury-related parkinsonism does not usually get worse over time and can stay stable over decades, whereas Parkinson's disease typically worsens gradually over time.

When to Refer: If you have addressed all of the issues above, and the signs and symptoms are clearly worsening over time, refer to a neurologist, ideally a movement disorders specialist, for evaluation and additional treatment.

21

Blurry Vision

Patients often complain that their vision is blurry or impaired in some way after concussion. Typically, this gets better on its own within a week to 2 weeks. However, if it doesn't, there are several possibilities. Ask the following questions and perform an examination at the same time:

(1) "Is it worse in one eye or the other? Or does it affect both eyes equally?" Perform visual acuity testing with the patient's corrective lenses using a near vision card with the right eye, left eye, then both eyes.
   a. A loss of acuity in one eye is often due to direct injury to the eye, which happens frequently in concussion. Refer to ophthalmology right away.
   b. Intact acuity in each eye, but worse vision with both eyes open is often due to a subtle cranial nerve injury. Subtle mismatch of eye movements can cause either double vision or blurry vision if the two images are very close together.
   c. Intact acuity in each eye individually and in both eyes together. Go on to the next questions.
(2) "Is it actually worse than before the injury?" Sometimes, patients will become aware of issues after concussion than were actually present beforehand. A collateral source will sometimes tell you something such as, "Oh, he's had 20/40 vision for years and never wanted to do anything about it." Refer to an optometrist. Patients will benefit from best corrected vision when starting aggressive cognitive rehabilitation, even if it didn't impair them much in everyday life before the concussion.

(3) "Is it worse when you look in one particular direction?" At the same time, ask the patient to follow your finger with their eyes up, down, left, and right. The goal is to determine whether there is a subtle cranial nerve deficit. Subtle third cranial nerve or fourth cranial injuries typically cause vision to be worse looking up or down, whereas sixth nerve injuries are typically worse looking to one side. Again, subtle mismatch of eye movements can cause either double vision or blurry vision if the two images are very close together. Even if you can't see a mismatch in the movement of the eyes, if there is a clear worsening of blurry vision or double vision with eye movement in one direction, it may be worthwhile to refer the patient to neuro-ophthalmology for a detailed evaluation and possibly for extraocular movement rehabilitation.

(4) "Is it OK in the morning but mainly a problem near the end of the day?" Visual attention deficit is sometimes described as blurry vision. Treat the attention deficit (Chapter 9).

(5) "Is it usually OK, but there are times when it gets much worse, sometimes followed by a bad headache?" Migraine auras often cause visual impairment of some kind: distorted vision, double vision, loss of central vision, loss of vision on one side of the visual world, sparkling lights, jagged lines, and so forth. Episodic changes in vision after concussion should be treated as presumptive migraine, or migraine equivalent even if there is not a severe headache (Chapter 7). Good migraine treatment can be very effective even if there is no headache.

(6) "Is it a problem with one kind of thing, like faces, or letters, or colors?" This is pretty rare after concussion but could indicate injury to a specific visual area in the brain. Obtain a magnetic resonance imaging (MRI) scan of the brain and refer to a cognitive neurologist. Often the scan will be negative, but specific rehabilitation can be helpful.

(7) None of the above. Unfortunately, some patients have impaired vision after concussion that doesn't fit any of

these patterns and is hard to understand. Sometimes it gets better on its own, and sometimes it does not, again for reasons that are not clear. It is possible that injury to higher visual pathways in the brain is responsible. Our current brain imaging technology isn't good enough to resolve subtle traumatic axonal injury in the optic nerve, optic radiations, thalamus, or cortex. Consider a referral to a neuro-ophthalmologist for a second opinion and re-examine the patient every 3 to 6 months to see if anything changes. Consider offering reassurance that there is not a serious cause of the blurry vision and refer the patient for a short course of occupational therapy for education in real world compensatory strategies. These cases are hard to interpret from a medico-legal standpoint.

22

Hearing Problems

The most common hearing problems after concussion are hypersensitivity to sound, tinnitus (ringing in the ears), and hearing loss. Military service members or others with blast-related concussion often have more than one of these problems.

Hypersensitivity to Sound (Hyperacusis)

Excessive sensitivity to sound can be due to migraine, damage to the ear and auditory nerve, or neuropathic pain. Whether it comes and goes versus stays stable does not seem to help determine the cause. A typical plan:

(1) Refer to an ear, nose, and throat (ENT) specialist for an evaluation of the middle and inner ear.

(2) Migraine pathophysiology can take many forms after concussion. As a therapeutic trial, offer treatment with an abortive migraine agent such as a triptan (e.g., "sumatriptan 50 mg po as soon as possible on onset of hypersensitive hearing") even if there is no accompanying headache. See the section on migraine for contraindications.

(3) As a therapeutic trial, offer treatment with a neuropathic pain agent such as pregabalin (Lyrica), carbamazepine (Tegretol), gabapentin (Neurontin), amitriptyline (Elavil), or oxcarbazepine (Trileptal). See the section on treatment of neuropathic-type headache in Chapter 7.

Tinnitus

Ringing or other noise in the ears after concussion can be disturbing to the patient, but it is rarely disabling. Often the specific cause of tinnitus cannot be identified. Consider treatment for attention deficit, migraine, and sleep dysfunction first. Tinnitus is most disturbing to patients who also have problems with attention, headache and sleep, so these interventions may make the tinnitus more tolerable. If it does not resolve, however, consider the following:

(1) Test hearing with an audiogram. If abnormal, refer to ENT for an evaluation of the middle and inner ear.
(2) Assess for medications that affect the inner ear, such as aminoglycoside antibiotics, aspirin, indomethacin, carbamazepine (Tegretol), propranolol (Inderal), levodopa (e.g., Sinemet), and caffeine. Consider the risk–benefit relationship and either stop the medication, lower the dose, or switch to a different medication for the same purpose.
(3) Test thyroid function.
(4) Order a magnetic resonance imaging (MRI) scan of the brain. Sometimes the concussion unmasks another unrelated problem such as an acoustic neuroma, arteriovenous malformation, or brainstem lesion. If the scan is normal, this is reassuring. It doesn't tell you what is causing the tinnitus, but it tells you that there aren't likely to be any big surprises.
(5) Refer to a specialized therapist team (audiologist and psychologist) for management training. A recent randomized (though not blinded) trial report indicated that 5 telephone-based sessions involving learning how to use therapeutic sound and cognitive behavioral therapy-based coping skills improved functional distress associated with tinnitus in both traumatic brain injury (TBI) patients and others (Henry et al, Ear & Hearing, 2018).

(6) Consider a small dose of a medication to try to suppress the tinnitus. None of these have been shown to be especially effective. Carefully evaluate whether there is a net benefit: Often the medications used to try to suppress tinnitus cause more cognitive dysfunction.
   a. Gabapentin (Neurontin) 300 mg po q6 hours
   b. Amitriptyline 25 mg po qhs
   c. Low-dose benzodiazepines such as diazepam (Valium) 1 to 2 mg po bid
(7) Consider referral to an ENT with specialty in tinnitus for advanced treatments.

Hearing Loss

A complaint of hearing loss can mean several things: true hearing loss due to middle or inner ear damage, attention deficit, or a language problem such as aphasia.

(1) Formally test hearing with an audiogram. If abnormal, refer to ENT for evaluation of the middle and inner ear and possible hearing aids.
(2) Assess for attention deficit and treat appropriately (Chapter 9).
(3) Assess for language problem: test naming of simple objects, repetition, and following commands. If there is a language problem, consider an MRI scan of the brain to evaluate for another cause in addition to concussion.

23

Smell and Taste Problems

Cranial nerve I, the olfactory nerve, is the most common peripheral nerve injured by head trauma. This is rarely the initial most significant complaint; often the patient will mention it on the second or third visit. There are two lines of treatment that may be worth pursuing. First, specialized rehabilitative strategies involving olfactory training can modestly improve smell perception. Olfactory rehabilitation training may only be available in specialized centers. However, the most important treatment is education for safety. Tell patients with severe loss of ability to smell (anosmia):

(1) You may not be aware of things burning in the house. Make sure all your smoke alarms are working well.
(2) You may not be aware of a natural gas leak in your house or office. Have someone else check periodically, or install a natural gas detector alarm (inexpensive and available at home improvement stores).
(3) You may not be aware of problems developing with your car, such as burning oil or leaking gasoline. Have someone else check it and keep a close eye on the dashboard lights every time you start up.
(4) You may not be able to tell if food has spoiled. Check expiration dates carefully, and if possible, have someone else taste the food if there is any doubt.
(5) You may find yourself eating too much because things taste bland and unsatisfying. Intensely spicy foods can bypass the olfactory system and stimulate the trigeminal nerve directly. This is one option for portion control: make your dishes spicier. Another option is to measure the portions,

eat slowly, and stop after you eat what you've measured, regardless of whether you feel satisfied or not.

A rare, but well-described complaint after partial loss of sense of smell is *phantosmia*, which means smelling things that aren't really there. The smells are often hard to describe exactly but are often quite unpleasant. No one knows for sure what causes this, but it is clearly real, and (despite the patient's worries), there is no evidence that it indicates patients are "going crazy." Treatment includes education and trials of medications usually used for neuropathic pain. This is based on the idea that perhaps the olfactory nerves are overactive as they are regrowing and that dampening down this overactivity will help address the phantosmia. Partial success has been reported with the following:

(1) Gabapentin (Neurontin) 300 mg po as needed up to 4 times per day (as for diabetic neuropathy).
(2) Carbamazepine (Tegretol) 200 mg po as needed up to 3 times per day (as for trigeminal neuralgia).
(3) Pregabalin (Lyrica) 50 mg po each evening or 50 mg bid (as for diabetic neuropathy).
(4) Venlafaxine (Effexor) 37.5 to 75 mg each day. Unclear why this would be helpful, but it has been reported to be.

24

Sexual Dysfunction

In private, ask specifically about sexual dysfunction, and if appropriate, ask the collateral source separately. Many patients will not mention it with the collateral source present, and a spouse or significant other may not bring it up with the patient present.

Take a systematic history

(1) Assess for depression (see Chapter 11) and treat if appropriate.

(2) Assess for severe fatigue or hypersomnia (see Chapters 16-17) and treat if appropriate.

(3) Check medications for sexual dysfunction as a side effect. Common offenders include:

    a. Selective serotonin reuptake inhibitors (SSRIs) such as citalopram (Celexa), escitalopram (Lexapro), fluoxetine (Prozac), paroxetine (Paxil), and sertraline (Zoloft). Consider switching to a serotonin–norepinephrine reuptake inhibitor (SNRI) such as venlafaxine (Effexor), bupropion (Wellbutrin), or trazodone. Anecdotally, amantadine has been reported to be helpful at relieving SSRI-related sexual dysfunction.

    b. Antipsychotics. For mood stabilization, consider switching to lamotrigine (Lamictal) or oxcarbazepine (Trileptal) (see Chapter 10).

    c. Narcotics. Consider switching to tramadol (Ultram) or nonsteroidal anti-inflammatories (ibuprofen, naproxen), and consider prescribing nonpharmacological approaches (see Chapters 7- 8).

    d. Propranolol. Consider switching to a calcium channel blocker or peripheral beta-blocker such as metoprolol or atenolol.

(4) Assess for untreated pain, either headaches or musculoskeletal.

(5) Assess for excess alcohol or illicit drug use, including marijuana.

    a. Large amounts of alcohol cause sexual dysfunction.

    b. Marijuana can cause sexual dysfunction in some people.

(6) Test for hormonal imbalances.

    a. In men, measure testosterone, thyroid-stimulating hormone, and cortisol.

    b. In women, measure estrogen, progesterone, thyroid-stimulating hormone, and cortisol.

(7) Assess for unrecognized spinal cord or cauda equina injury.

    a. Ask about urinary incontinence, loss of perineal sensation, leg weakness or numbness.

    b. Check knee and ankle reflexes.

        i. Very brisk reflexes can indicate spinal cord compression. Consider a cervical and thoracic spine magnetic resonance imaging (MRI) scan to evaluate for spinal cord compression.

        ii. Absent reflexes can indicate nerve root injury. Consider a lumbar and sacral spine MRI to evaluate the cauda equina.

        iii. Refer to neurosurgery if the scans are abnormal.

If none of the above are present, consider nonspecific treatment.

(1) Phosphodiesterase type 5 (PDE5) inhibitors for men (and possibly for women, though less direct evidence).

    a. Sildenafil (Viagra): 25 to 100 mg po 30 minutes before sexual activity.

      b. Tadalafil (Cialis): 5 to 20 mg po with more flexible timing, before sexual activity or daily.

      c. Contraindications include use of nitrates or alpha blockers such as prazosin, due to risk of hypotension.

      d. No specific contraindication following concussion.

(2) Refer to a urologist for more advanced assessments and treatments.

25

Seizures

Concussion rarely causes recurrent seizures. People commonly have one or two brief (< 1 min) seizures within the first few minutes after the concussion, but this does not mean that the person has epilepsy or is at elevated risk for future seizures. *A patient with a seizure that occurs within the first 30 minutes of concussion does not need to be treated with antiepileptics.* The patient does not automatically need to have driving privileges revoked or need to be put on other restrictions such as swimming or bathing alone, working at heights, operating machinery. However, a seizure occurring later than 30 minutes after the injury, a seizure that lasts more than 1 minute, or a seizure after concussion in a patient with a previous seizure disorder requires a different approach (see Figure 25.1).

(1) Was it really a seizure? Syncope can also cause brief convulsions.
(2) Early, brief, uncomplicated seizures don't require treatment. Did the seizure have all of the following characteristics :
   a. Occurred within 30 minutes of concussion
   b. Lasted less than 1 minute
   c. Patient had no previous seizure disorder.

If so, no additional evaluation or treatment is needed. Observe as for concussion in general.

   If not, go to *Evaluation and Treatment*

(3) Evaluation of late or prolonged seizure after concussion
   a. Observe carefully in the hospital for at least 24 hours.

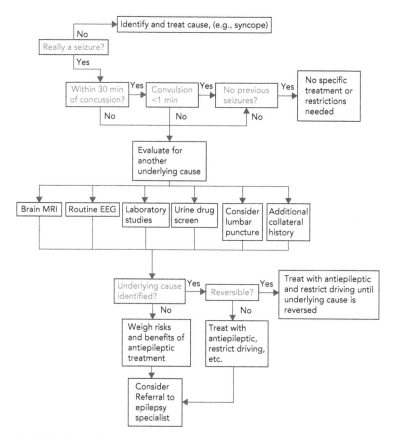

FIGURE 25.1 Seizures after concussion.

b. Obtain a magnetic resonance imaging (MRI) scan of the brain with and without contrast to make sure there is not a more serious injury or another underlying structural brain lesion that was "unmasked" by the concussion.

c. Obtain a routine electroencephalogram (EEG) to rule out focal abnormalities that suggest an underlying brain structural lesion. Sleep deprivation is not recommended.

d. Lab studies: complete blood count (CBC) looking for infection; comprehensive metabolic panel (CMP) looking for electrolyte or metabolic dysfunction.

e. Consider lumbar puncture if any sign of central nervous system (CNS) infection: fever, neck stiffness, mental status change preceding the concussion. This is important—sometimes a CNS infection such as herpes simplex encephalitis can cause abnormal behavior, which then leads to a fall or motor vehicle crash.

f. Urine drug screen

g. Careful history from a reliable collateral source regarding

    i. Alcohol use and possible abrupt withdrawal.

    ii. Illicit drug use (not everything shows up on the drug screen).

    iii. Prescription drug use and possible abrupt withdrawal.

    iv. Recent sleep deprivation.

(4) Treatment principles

a. If there is an obvious cause that can be fixed, fix it. If the cause can be fully reversed, it is not necessary to treat with an antiepileptic.

b. If there is an obvious cause that cannot be fully reversed, then treat with an antiepileptic medication.

c. If there is no obvious cause, it's a judgment call. Consider the risks and benefits (pros and cons) of treating with an antiepileptic.

    i. PRO: may reduce risk of future seizures (probably true, but no actual evidence for this).

    ii. CON: may cause side effects, expense, and inconvenience.

d. Choice of antiepileptics:

    i. Maximize compliance and minimize side effects. All of the medications are equally effective (or ineffective), but they differ a lot in terms of side effects.

        1. This means probably NOT phenytoin (Dilantin), valproic acid (Depakote), or phenobarbital (substantial side effects).

    ii. Mood stabilization is better than destabilization

1. Prefer oxcarbazepine (Trileptal), lamotrigine (Lamictal), or carbamazepine (Tegretol) over levetiracetam (Keppra), which can be mood destabilizing.
2. Lamotrigine (Lamictal) appears to have the least cognitive side effects and is mood stabilizing. But it takes a long time to get to therapeutic dose.
3. A common plan is to use an oxcarbazepine bridge to lamotrigine:

a. Oxcarbazepine 300 mg po bid x 7 days, then 600 mg po bid x 2 months
b. Lamotrigine starter kit starting right away. Starts with 25 mg each day then increasing every 2 weeks until 100 mg bid over 2 months.
c. Lamotrigine 200 mg po bid and stop oxcarbazepine after 2 months.

4. Carbamazepine generic often the best choice when cost is an issue.

26

Psychosis

New onset hallucinations and delusions are pretty rare after concussion. These symptoms should trigger a search for other causes, primarily by history obtained from the collateral source:

(1) Prior psychotic disorder exacerbated by the concussion. Approximately 1% of the general population has schizophrenia, and it often presents in adolescence and early adulthood, around the age when people are doing risky things that lead to concussion.

(2) Drug abuse or toxic substances: Psychosis can be triggered by amphetamines, cocaine, LSD, PCP, hallucinogenic mushrooms, ecstasy, and many other drugs. We've seen several cases of psychosis caused by marijuana laced with other substances. Take a careful history and get a urine drug screen.

(3) Prescription drug effects and drug–drug interactions. Narcotic pain medications are the most common offenders.

(4) Alcohol or benzodiazepine withdrawal

(5) Endocrine disorder: check for hyperthyroidism and hypocortisolemia with a thyroid-stimulating hormone (TSH) and morning cortisol level.

(6) Make sure it is really psychosis, and not delirium (waxing and waning level of arousal), which can also be accompanied by hallucinations and delusions. Delirium has a very long differential diagnosis. Most notably sleep deprivation, urinary tract infections in the elderly, and poly-pharmacy with multiple central nervous system acting medications.

Importantly, if the psychosis is dangerous or potentially dangerous, think about safety first. This may require admission to a psychiatric ward for a few days to let things settle down.

Pharmacological treatment: Usually with an atypical antipsychotic. This is different from acute onset of psychosis from other causes in that often, lower doses of antipsychotics are effective, and cognitive side effects of medication can be especially troublesome.

(1) No clear preference for one over the other in terms of efficacy.

(2) Aripiprazole (Abilify): 1 to 2 mg qhs. Often chosen because it is associated with less weight gain than other antipsychotics.

(3) Risperidone (Risperdal): 0.5 to 1 mg bid is the least expensive.

(4) Quetiapine (Seroquel): 5 to 10 mg bid, or rarely Clozaril, are the best choices when parkinsonism is a comorbidity, as often occurs as a chronic degenerative condition after multiple concussions (likely part of chronic traumatic encephalopathy).

In the short term, monitor for akathisia (restlessness), weight gain, parkinsonism (resting tremor, slowness of movement, and stiffness), and cognitive impairment. If these are intolerable, reduce the dose or switch to a different agent.

In the long-term, monitor for tardive dyskinesia (involuntary twisting, writhing movements). If this is troublesome, reduce the dose and refer to a movement disorders center or a psychiatrist with expertise in this area.

27

Return to Work

This is one of the hardest problems facing the provider caring for patients with complex concussions. Every case is different. A lot depends on the nature of the work. The criteria are quite different for a long-haul truck driver or law enforcement officer than for an office worker. It is important to get this right the first time, because often if the patient tries to go back to work too soon and makes a serious error, he or she may lose the job and never get another chance to try again. Give an honest prognosis with a positive spin. Avoid the "nocebo" effect that comes from setting an expectation of sickness. Most people recover well from concussion and return to work.

In general, follow these principles:

(1) The patient should receive optimal treatment for headaches, sleep disorders, fatigue, anxiety, depression, mood instability, and attention deficit before attempting to return to work. Any of these, if untreated, can result in poor performance at work.

(2) An occupational therapist should try to simulate the patient's workplace or most important work-related tasks to see how the patient performs, then attempt to develop compensatory strategies. Ideally, this should be done by a specialized occupational performance center. The therapists should come out to the patient's workplace to see firsthand what the patient's work entails.

(3) Start back to work slowly if the patient has been out of work for more than a month. For example:
  a. Half day on Monday, Wednesday, and Friday the first week, then
  b. 5 half days the second week, then

    c. 3 full days the third week, then
    d. Full time the fourth week.

The patient should keep going to occupational therapy during the transition to address any real-world deficits that become apparent and may not have been noticed beforehand. It is common for migraine headaches, mood instability, and attention deficit to manifest more clearly during the first attempt to return to work.

(4) Be more conservative with patients in high-risk occupations such as professional drivers, law enforcement personnel, active duty military with potential combat duties, or heavy equipment operators.
    a. Communicate directly with the patient's supervisor to make sure you understand the workplace requirements.
    b. Ask whether there is any "light duty" that the patient can do as part of the rehabilitation process.
    c. Make sure that the patient is closely watched during a transition period lasting between 1 week and 1 year after return to work.

(5) For patients in high cognitive demand professions, tell the patient and collateral source that his or her abilities may not be back to 100% right away, and advise him or her not to make any major decisions or take on any major new responsibilities right away. Advise the patient to do everything he or she had been doing well before taking on anything new. Some high-functioning patients who were pushing their cognitive limits prior to concussion may have to return to work at a lower level. The concept of cognitive reserve helps explain this. Even when the patient has made what seems like a good recovery, there can be some loss of cognitive reserve. Patients who were not using their cognitive abilities at work to the maximum potential may not notice the loss of reserve. But for those who are pushing right to the edge, it may be more apparent.

There is not yet a clear evidence base for interventions to improve return-to-work success.

Resource facilitation services provided over a 15-month period modestly improved the rate and timing of return to productive community-based work compared to control in a mixed group of acquired brain injury patients, but very few had concussion as their primary injury (Trexler et al, Archives of Physical and Rehabilitation Medicine, 2016).

A recent randomized controlled trial of a 5-session cognitive behavioral therapy intervention versus telephone counseling after concussion revealed similar return-to-work outcomes (Scheenen et al, Journal of Neurotrauma, 2017). Somewhat surprisingly, the group receiving telephone counseling involving 5 phone conversations starting 4 to 6 weeks after injury had fewer complaints and a higher likelihood of full recovery at 12 months than the cognitive behavioral therapy group.

Similarly, a randomized controlled trial of intensive outpatient management and education versus routine general practitioner follow-up did not reveal a significant difference in return-to-work outcomes after concussion, though there was some reduction in symptoms in the intensive outpatient management group (Vikane et al, Brain Injury, 2017).

28

Return to Driving

Most concussion patients can return to driving without any problems at around the same time they return to work or school. In complex concussion patients, however, it is not always clear whether it is safe for the patient to return to driving. In a recent study, some concussion patients were found to have impaired driving simulator performance even after they had become entirely symptom-free (Schmidt et al, Journal of Neurotrauma, 2017). The patient may not be aware of his or her own deficits, and the collateral source may not want to irritate the patient by pointing out these deficits in public. A family member may say something like, "I didn't want to say this in front of him, but I'm really worried about whether it is safe for him to drive—he gets so irritable behind the wheel." The risk is serious; the patient may have an accident and reinjure his or her brain before it has fully healed, injure someone else, or damage a vehicle.

Return to driving requires the practitioner to make a judgment, based on a combination of the law, medical knowledge, and a bit of insight (see Figure 28.1).

A. Assess for definite contraindications to driving.

(1) Seizure disorder (Laws vary by region; in most places the patient has to be seizure free for 6 to 12 months.)
(2) Other cause of intermittent unpredictable loss of consciousness (e.g., cardiac arrhythmia)
(3) Severe hypersomnolence
(4) Performance-impairing medications
(5) Visual impairment
(6) Psychosis

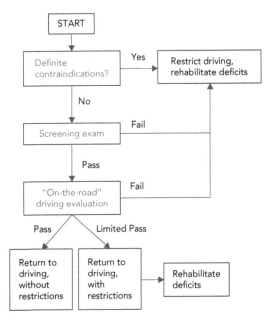

FIGURE 28.1 Driving after concussion.

(7) Severe impulsivity
(8) Poor decision-making
(9) Obvious physical impairment

If it is not safe for the patient to drive because of one or more of these contraindications, write this down on a prescription and give it to the collateral source so that there are no arguments about what was said in the office visit. Then refer the patient to occupational therapy to address the concern if possible.

B. If there are no obvious definite contraindications to driving, perform the following *screening exam*:

(1) Test visual acuity with both eyes open and best corrective lenses. Visual acuity should be 20/40 or better.

(2) Test peripheral vision by asking the patient to count fingers flashed in all 4 quadrants. http://www.youtube.com/watch?v=XiEw7v7OyBw

(3) Test for visual neglect by asking the patient to count fingers flashed in both the left and right upper quadrants at the same time, then left and right lower quadrants.

(4) Test saccades: rapid eye movements to each of the 4 directions ("look at my nose, now look quickly at my finger"). Very slow or inaccurate saccades may make driving unsafe.

(5) Head turn side to side. The patient should be able to look over his or her shoulder, as if changing lanes.

(6) Rapid alternating hand movements.

(7) Rapid foot movements (tap your right foot as fast as you can).

(8) Orientation to location and approximate time of day.

(9) Visuospatial memory: Hide 3 objects around the office, then ask the patient to find them 5 minutes later, with the above tests as distracters in between. Even if verbal memory is poor, visuospatial memory may be intact. If it is not, the patient may still be able to drive but only with someone else along, to prevent the patient from getting lost.

If the patient fails any of these screening tests, refer to occupational therapy or physical therapy to rehabilitate the deficits if possible and readdress the question of driving on the patient's next visit. Write down the reason for restricting driving on a prescription and give it to the collateral source to prevent any arguments about what was said.

C. If the patient passes all of the parts of the screening exam, refer him or her for an *"on-the-road" driving evaluation* performed by a specialized service. This is typically expensive (from $200 to $300 in St. Louis, Missouri) and may not be covered by insurance. Tell the patient that it is a lot less expensive than having an accident. If patients pass the on-the-road test, they may return to driving. If they fail the on-the-road test, refer to occupational therapy or physical therapy to attempt to rehabilitate the deficits that caused the failure. Impulsivity is a common reason for failure after concussion. This can be treated by occupational therapy.

D. Specialty vehicle drivers will require an even more careful evaluation. Direct observation by the supervisor will be required.

29

Return to School

Returning to school is harder than returning to work in many cases. At work, the patient can usually go back to doing things he or she already knows how to do. At school, the patient is expected to learn new things every day.

Consider a graded, stepwise approach, analogous to the strategy for return to play (see Figure 29.1). This requires coordination with teachers, administrators, school nursing/medical providers, parents, and often classmates (Halstead et al., *Pediatrics*, 2013). Again, give an honest prognosis with a positive spin. Avoid the "no-cebo" effect that comes from setting an expectation of sickness. Most people recover well from concussion and return to school.

The approach depends on whether the patient had an acute, relatively straightforward concussion, or a more complex concussion scenario (e.g., a second concussion before full recovery from the first, concussion complicated by severe migraine, or chronic concussion-related symptoms).

> *There is no scientific evidence to support the specific details of this approach; many versions are possible.*

Some flexibility with the specific times and accommodations is recommended. Results of a recent study suggest that reduced cognitive activity is associated with faster resolution of concussion-related symptoms, but that complete cognitive rest is not necessary (Brown et al., *Pediatrics*, 2014).

Some patients can move through this progression faster, especially after more minor concussions with no residual symptoms at all after 24 hours.

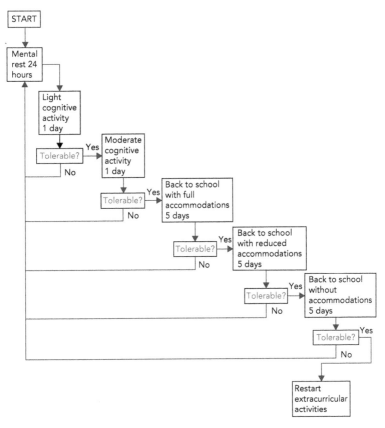

FIGURE 29.1 Return to school after typical concussion.

Acutely after a Substantial but Relatively Straightforward Concussion

(Step 1) *Mental rest* for 24 hours. No homework, no reading, no text messages, nothing. Parents or classmates should contact teachers and administrators to arrange this, so that the concussed person does not get stressed out. *Typically, emergency departments or primary care providers provide this guidance.*

(Step 2) Light cognitive activity: for example, reading *familiar material* for 20 minutes, no more. If the patient can't tolerate the full 20 minutes, then go back to Step 1. If the patient can do 20 minutes with at most some tolerable exacerbation of symptoms, rest for at least 30 minutes or until any worsening of headache, fatigue, blurry vision, mood instability, or other symptoms brought on by the light cognitive activity has resolved. This could take until the next day. Then move to Step 3.

(Step 3) Moderate cognitive activity: for example, 50 minutes of *new material* in a class that is relatively easy—often the student's strongest subject. This could involve catching up on one lesson or one homework assignment that was missed due to the concussion. If this is intolerable, then go back to Step 1. If the patient can do 50 minutes with at most some tolerable exacerbation of symptoms, rest for at least 60 minutes, or until any worsening of headache, fatigue, blurry vision, mood instability, or other symptoms brought on by the moderate cognitive activity has resolved. This could take until the next day. Then move to Step 4.

(Step 4) Back to school with the following accommodations for the first 5 school days:

- No tests for 2 to 3 weeks, justified as follows: The symptoms are expected to clear within 7 to 10 days, and then the patient will need at least 1 full week to study and catch up on the material that was missed.
- Rest breaks as needed during the school day. The teachers and the school nurse or other medical providers should all understand that the patient may need one or several 15- to 30-minute rest breaks during the day.
- No homework for 5 school days in the patient's single most challenging subject. After concussion, this is often math. This break allows the patient to get back into school and get most of the way caught up without getting overly fatigued mentally.

- No extracurricular activities such as sports, clubs, or performing arts unless these are critical to future career plans or of great value to the patient.
- Rest 1 extra hour each afternoon, and sleep 1 extra hour each night.
- Go to bed and wake up at the same time on weekend nights as during the week. No late night or early morning social activities.

If symptoms and signs become intolerable, go all the way back to step 2 and make an appointment with a concussion specialist—this may not be a smooth recovery. The appointment can be cancelled if the patient recovers again quickly. If a concussion specialist is not available, begin treatment of the most disabling specific symptoms (most typically headache, attention deficit, and mood instability). If symptoms do not recur, or recur but are tolerable, move on to Step 5. Importantly, it is expected for patients to have some subjectively experienced or objectively observed impairment in cognitive performance this week, but it should be improving steadily day by day. It is also expected for patients to have some recurrence of moderate symptoms. Most symptom "spikes" resolve within 24 hours. You do not have to go back to Step 1 for every symptom. Stated another way, the patient does not have to be completely asymptomatic to move to the next step.

(Step 5) Back to school with homework in all classes during the second week but otherwise same accommodations as the first week. If symptoms become intolerable go back to Step 2 and make an appointment with a concussion specialist. Importantly, cognitive performance should be normal at this point. If the patient is having cognitive performance concerns, go back to Step 2 and make an appointment with a concussion specialist.

(Step 6) Back to school with no accommodations during the third week. Catch up on missed tests and homework.

(Step 7) Restart extracurricular activities AFTER all the academic work is caught up.

In addition to symptoms, carefully assess for executive function problems. These can include issues with organization and planning, working memory, initiation, monitoring one's own progress, impulse control, transitioning from one activity to the next, responding appropriately, anticipating future events, and keeping track of the effects of one's own behavior on others. Problems with executive function can be a big impediment to successful return to school. They are not always obvious right away. Take a careful history from parents and teachers. Consider using a quantitative measure such as the Behavior Rating Inventory of Executive Function (BRIEF), which is based on a very well validated set of questions for parents and teachers that takes about 10 to 15 minutes to administer on paper or online. There is a small charge for the test. https://www.parinc.com/Products/Pkey/23.

Back to School Form for Patients and Families

Date and Time of Concussion:			
Date	Step	Symptoms	Tolerable?
	Mental Rest		

More Complex Concussions

Return to school in patients with complex concussion may take longer (see Figure 29.2). This may include, for example, patients who have been out of school for weeks, patients who have tried to return to school and been unable to do so, or patients with very severe symptoms or a history of many previous concussions.

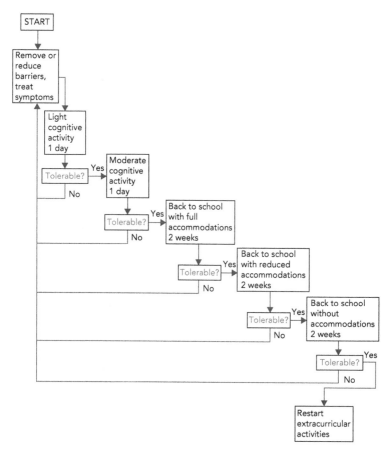

FIGURE 29.2 Return to school after complex concussion.

(Step 1) Remove or reduce as many of the barriers to optimal cognitive performance as possible. At a minimum, treat sleep disorders, headache, depression, and anxiety to get symptoms down to tolerable levels. There is no point in trying to return to school when any of these are severe enough to be disabling or substantially impairing. This may take 4 to 6 weeks. Treat hearing and vision impairments optimally. During this time, the patient should do very light cognitive activity; for example, reading enjoyable material for 20 minutes at a time, then resting for at least 30 minutes or until any exacerbation of symptoms has resolved. Some light cardiovascular exercise such as walking for 30 to 60 minutes a day as tolerated can be helpful to prevent deconditioning and improve sleep.

(Step 2) Light cognitive activity: for example, reading familiar material for 20 minutes, no more. If the patient can't do the full 20 minutes, then take 1 full day of cognitive rest and try again. Regardless of how it goes, rest for at least 30 minutes, or until any worsening of headache, fatigue, blurry vision, or other symptoms brought on by the light cognitive activity has resolved. This could take until the next day.

(Step 3) Moderate cognitive activity: for example, 50 minutes of new material in a class that is relatively easy—the student's strongest subject. This could involve catching up on 1 lesson or 1 homework assignment that was missed due to the concussion. If the patient can't do the full 50 minutes, then take 1 full day of cognitive rest and try again. Regardless of how it goes, rest for at least 60 minutes, or until any worsening of headache, fatigue, blurry vision, or other symptoms brought on by the moderate cognitive activity has resolved. This could take until the next day.

(Step 4) Make a plan with school administrators, teachers, parents, classmates, and others for a trial of returning to school. This has to be agreeable to everyone involved, so it will need to be individualized. Some flexibility with regard to the specific details will be required.

An example: Back to school with accommodations

Weeks 1 and 2

- No tests, justified as follows: adaptation is expected to take 4 weeks, and then the patient will need at least 2 full weeks to study and catch up on the material that was missed.
- Rest breaks as needed during the school day. The teachers and the school nurse or other medical provider should all understand that the patient may need one or several 15- to 30-minute rest breaks during the day.
- No homework for 2 weeks in the patient's single most challenging subject. After concussion, this is often math. This allows the patient to get back into school and get most of the way caught up without getting overly mentally fatigued.
- No extracurricular activities such as sports, clubs, or performing arts.
- Rest 1 extra hour each afternoon, sleep 1 extra hour each night. If the patient falls asleep late and wakes up late, allow the patient to come to school 1 hour later than the normal start time.
- Go to bed and wake up at the same time on weekend nights as during the week. No late night or early morning social activities.

Weeks 3 and 4

Restart homework in the most challenging subject, while otherwise maintaining the same accommodations.

Weeks 5 and 6

Catch up on all missed homework and make up missed tests. Rest breaks during these makeup tests could be appropriate.

Restart extracurricular activities *AFTER* all the academic work is caught up, no earlier than Week 7.

An alternative, even more conservative approach would be to return to school half time for the rest of the semester and make up the dropped classes in the summer. This could be appropriate if the major symptoms, such as headaches, depression, anxiety, insomnia, and attention deficit are proving refractory to first-line treatment.

A final, extremely conservative approach would be to recommend taking just a single class with the understanding that the patient probably will not graduate on time. This is rarely appropriate after concussion, but more often is required after more severe traumatic brain injury (TBI). It is still better than not returning to school at all.

30

Return to Contact Sports

There are several sets of published guidelines on this topic, which apply generally to simple concussions. Please see McCrory et al., *British Journal of Sports Medicine*, 2017 for the 2016 Berlin consensus statement on concussion in sport.

Rule 1) No return to play in the same 24-hour period as the concussion.

Rule 2) Graded, stepwise increases in activity guided by symptoms.

Rule 3) No difference in return to play for elite versus nonelite athletes.

Rule 4) Brief convulsions or posturing at the time of concussion does not indicate higher than normal risk of seizures and requires no specific management.

Rule 5) The player should not be left alone after the injury and should be monitored frequently for the first few hours.

None of these recommendations, however, cover what to do with patients whose concussions are more complex—those who haven't recovered with the graded resumption-of-activity approach outlined in Figure 30.1 and in the Berlin 2016 consensus statement.

In some cases, extra time is all that is needed. Recent studies have shown that 10 to 14 days for adults and up to 4 weeks for children is the most common timeline for full recovery. This is longer than the 6- to 10-day period initially believed. Among collegiate athletes, females recover a bit slower than males on average, and club/intramural athletes recover more slowly than varsity athletes.

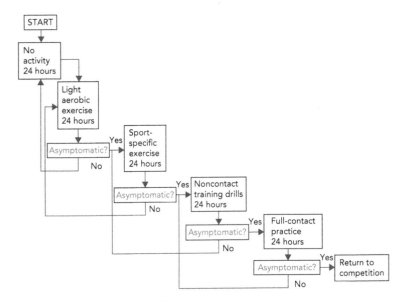

FIGURE 30.1 Return to play after typical concussion.

After 2 weeks in adults and 4 weeks in children, more rest is not likely to help. At that point, it is reasonable to start active interventions.

Severe migraine, early symptoms of depression, and numerous troubling symptoms are all clues that the patient may not get better with just rest, and active interventions are going to be required (see Figure 30.2).

(1) The first question is whether the patient should return to sports at all. Consider letting the patient make his or her own decision, but provide the patient with appropriate information on which to base this decision using the following process. Make sure that the patient has really thought it through logically. Consider asking these questions:

a. "Are you going to be a professional athlete?"

b. "Are you interested in a career that requires thinking, memory, or good interpersonal relationships? There is

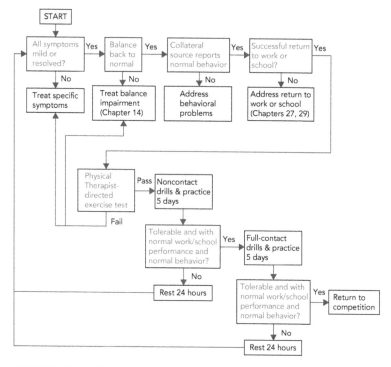

FIGURE 30.2 Return to play after complex concussion.

some risk that multiple concussions will permanently impair your abilities in these areas."

c. "Are there any other types of exercise that you can do that involve a lower risk of head injury?"

For most patients, their long-term well-being depends more on their work and interpersonal relationships than on their athletic performance. After thinking it through carefully, many patients will decide on their own not to return to contact sports. For most people, it's just not worth it.

In 3 instances strong advice about not returning to sport can be given:

a. *Full contact combative sports such as professional boxing and mixed martial arts. After a complex concussion from* which the patient is not making a rapid and complete recovery, consider strongly advising combative sport athletes to retire. The risk of further concussions is very high, and the potential long-term adverse effects are well-documented. In these cases, consider administering a big dose of "Vitamin S" (the therapeutic scare) by telling the patient and collateral source about the possible long-term effects of multiple concussions, such as chronic traumatic encephalopathy.

b. *Extreme sports with a high risk of death or permanent injury if there is an error in judgment, timing, or coordination.* High-altitude mountaineering, base jumping, backcountry skiing, ski racing, motorcycle racing, and bullfighting fall into this category.

c. *The patient is on anticoagulants.* In these cases, the risk of major bleeding in the brain is substantially elevated. The patient should not return to contact sports.

(2) Discourage the patient from returning to contact sports until *all* of the following are true:

a. The symptoms are all in the tolerable range or resolved AND

b. The collateral source verifies that the patient's behavior is back to normal AND

c. The patient has been able to successfully return to school or work (for nonprofessional athletes), AND

d. Balance is back to baseline (if known), or back to normal if baseline is not known. The Balance Error Scoring System (BESS) is recommended for this assessment.

(3) If the patient's symptoms, behavior, school/work performance, and balance are normal or near normal at rest and tolerable with light activity, prescribe a physical therapist-directed moderate exercise test. The therapist will direct the patient to exercise in clinic (going up and down stairs, doing squats, pushups, standing jumps, etc.) to get the patient's heart rate over 70% of predicted maximum for at least 5 minutes. Then assess the patient's symptoms again

using the Rivermead postconcussive symptoms questionnaire, test balance using the BESS, and perform another neurological exam.

If symptoms become intolerable or balance substantially deteriorates after moderate exercise, go back to Step 1 and retest after the specific concern has been addressed (e.g., medication treatment for headaches, physical therapy balance training for balance).

If symptoms are tolerable and balance remains stable after moderate exercise, advance to noncontact drills and practice for 1 week (Step 4).

(4) Non-contact drills and practice for 1 week. Write a note and contact the patient's coach and trainer to make sure that the plan is communicated clearly. Some patients will tell the coach that they are clear, without restrictions. If patient tolerates noncontact drills and practice for 1 week without recurrence of symptoms or deterioration of balance and is still able to maintain good performance in work or school, advance to full contact drills and practice. If the patient deteriorates with noncontact drills and practice, go back to Step 1.

(5) Full contact drills and practice but no competition for 1 week. Again, write a note and contact the patient's coach and trainer to make sure that the plan is communicated clearly. If patient tolerates full contact drills and practice for 1 week without recurrence of symptoms or deterioration of balance and is still able to maintain good performance in work or school, advance to competition. If the patient deteriorates with noncontact drills and practice, go back to Step 1.

Another approach to exercise testing is based on the Buffalo Concussion Treadmill Test. http://www.biact.org/assets/uploads/files/Conference/Annual%20Conference%20Archives/Buffalo%20Concussion%20Treadmill%20Test%20Manual%20-%20edits.pdf

This test is recommended for athletes who have had symptoms for more than 3 weeks after concussion. The goal is to figure out whether the athlete can return to moderate exercise. The athlete exercises on a treadmill under supervision until significant symptom exacerbation. The maximum heart rate is recorded. The authors of the Buffalo Concussion Treadmill Test recommend that the athlete can be given a prescription for 20 minutes of daily cardiovascular exercise not to exceed 80% of the maximum heart rate reached without significant symptom exacerbation. So far, this protocol seems to be safe in patients without cardiovascular contraindications to exercise. If maximum exertion is reached without significant symptom exacerbation, the authors of the Buffalo Concussion Treadmill Test recommend that the athlete can go on to the Zurich consensus plan involving graded, stepwise increases in activity guided by symptoms over approximately 6 to 10 days, just like after an acute concussion (Leddy et al., Current Sports Medicine Reports, 2013).

Neck Strengthening: If the patient decides to return to sports, consider recommending extra neck-strengthening exercises. There is some evidence that a stronger more muscular neck reduces the extent of rotational acceleration of the head and may provide some protection from concussion (Jin et al., Journal of Biomechanical Engineering, 2017). Athletes in many sports and military personnel may already be doing these exercises. They may be especially beneficial for athletes who have slimmer or weaker necks. The flip side is that a very large, muscular neck puts the patient at high risk of obstructive sleep apnea. Discuss the pros and cons of neck strengthening with the patient.

If the patient does return to sports and has another concussion or recurrence of symptoms, consider recommending a longer-than-normal rest period. For example, 7 days of full rest then graded return to normal activity. This can be the "wake-up call" that gets the patient to change sports.

When Is It Safe to Fly or Travel to High Altitude?

Most commercial airplanes are pressurized to the equivalent of about 7000 to 8000 feet. U.S. Air Force researchers have shown that uninjured people experience very little change in cognitive function or symptoms at this altitude, but this is not the case after concussion. Symptoms and deficits that had resolved can come back at altitude, most notably headaches, slowing of cognitive performance, and impaired balance. Inform the patient and family about this risk and then let them make their own decisions about whether it is worth it. No evidence of permanent harm from flying or traveling to moderate altitude in concussion patients exists, but it has not been carefully studied.

Medico-legal Aspects of Concussion

Many patients involved in a motor vehicle accident, workplace injury, or assault will have a lawsuit or criminal action pending at the time you see them in clinic. When the patient and family have a lot to gain financially from the outcome of the legal action, the question arises about whether their symptoms and disabilities are being reported accurately or magnified for the purposes of secondary gain. To answer this question, *reliable and unbiased collateral source information is critical*. Under most circumstances, a family member may be an ideal collateral source, but when there is a legal action pending, the collateral sources should be people who know the patient well before and after the injury but don't have a financial stake one way or another in the outcome. Often, coworkers, neighbors, or community leaders are good choices. It can be a lot of work to find the right collateral sources. It is not wrong to have the patient sit in the exam room while you call people on the phone. Sometimes you won't have all the information you need until the collateral source calls you back. Again, it is reasonable to start treating the patient and make the final diagnosis later. On the whole, patients' quality of life is helped more by treating their symptoms effectively than by winning a lawsuit.

Most people who have been at their jobs for many years and like them are not likely to consider a lawsuit for secondary gain. But even people with a less-than-rock-solid work history can have persistent impairments from concussions and be involved in lawsuits without necessarily being interested in secondary gain. Again, this takes time, collateral source information, and a bit of insight to sort out.

It is worth reiterating here that no scan or test can "rule in" or "rule out" concussion. Typically, computed tomography (CT) scans and magnetic resonance imaging (MRI) scans are normal, and there will not be any "objective" evidence for concussion. Thus, the history obtained from reliable and unbiased collateral sources represents the best available evidence.

There is one exception: In the acute phase after concussion, if you think there is a high likelihood that there will be a medico-legal case, it is worthwhile to get an MRI scan with susceptibility weighted imaging on as powerful a scanner as you can access (e.g., 3T better than 1.5T, closed better than open). These acute phase MRI scans are more likely to show small hemorrhages in character-istic locations such as the junction of cortical gray matter and white matter or corpus callosum than MRI scans performed later. If the scan is positive, it makes the medico-legal case a lot easier. If it is negative or nonspecific, it still doesn't rule out concussion, it just doesn't help with the medico-legal case and you are back to collat-eral source information.

Incarcerated criminals are at very high risk of sustaining concussions while in custody, and a substantial proportion have a prior history of brain injury. There is emerging evidence that con-cussion and other brain injuries put criminals at higher risk of re-arrest after they have been released from custody. Social workers or other health care coordinators should be involved to make sure that incarcerated and recently released criminals receive appro-priate medical care, get to their appointments, comply with lifestyle recommendations, and are able to fill medication prescriptions.

33

Concussion in the Elderly

Elderly individuals over age 65 represent the fastest growing group of traumatic brain injury patients. In many parts of the world, the rates of concussion in the elderly now exceed the rates in adolescents. Most of these injuries are due to falls. Although subdural hemorrhage after falls has long been the "hallmark" injury in this population, concussive injuries without intracranial hemorrhage are far more common. Thus, the same rule applies; a negative scan does not rule out concussion.

Special Management Considerations

(1) Many elderly individuals are taking anticoagulant medications, and an initial computed tomography (CT) scan is warranted to rule out intracranial hemorrhage. Recent evidence, however, indicates that a second CT scan is generally unnecessary if the first scan is negative and the patient's neurological condition is stable (Campiglio et al., Neurology. Clinical Practice, 2017).

(2) Elderly can be more susceptible to the anticholinergic side effects of medications. Typically, tricyclic antidepressants such as amitriptyline should be used at lower doses or avoided.

(3) Elderly can be more susceptible to the other side effects of medications. Again, smaller doses may be preferred initially. Stimulants may be poorly tolerated due to cardiovascular and cerebrovascular concerns, so acetylcholinesterase inhibitors

may be preferred for attention deficits even though they are less effective.

(4) Physical therapy treatment for fall prevention is recommended to reduce the risk of additional concussions.

(5) Balance training such as yoga, tai chi, and dance may also reduce the risk of additional concussions.

(6) Concussion is associated with increased risk of subsequent dementia. The order of causality, however, cannot be determined precisely—injury could accelerate dementia, or the event leading to the injury could have been due to previously underappreciated cognitive impairment. Nonetheless, vigilance with regard to progressive cognitive decline is warranted.

(7) Concussion is associated with increased risk of subsequent Parkinson's disease. Again, the order of causality cannot be determined precisely and vigilance with regard to progressive worsening of motor function is warranted.

(8) Driving may be especially problematic in elderly. Special efforts should be made to ensure that elderly patients can safely make it to their therapy appointments (e.g., ride services, taxis, family, friends, or public transit). A prescription for home-based therapy services may be more appropriate.

34

Concussion in Adolescents

In general, most aspects of concussion in 13- to 18-year-olds are similar to those in adults, with the following exceptions:

(1) The patient may be less able to make good judgments about his or her own abilities than an adult. The collateral source becomes even more important than usual. The patient may not remember accurately how severe the headaches were 2 weeks ago if he or she feels OK today. The patient may deny problems with attention and concentration but be doing poorly in school. Strongly consider obtaining additional collateral-source information from a teacher.

> *On the other hand, some adolescents are extraordinarily mature and can be treated just like adults. The concept of the "mature minor" has made it through the legal system in several U.S. states, and the conclusion has been that a "mature" (as evaluated jointly by the physician and collateral sources) minor should have full decision-making authority.*

(2) The patient may not want his or her parents to know about use of drugs and alcohol. Ask these questions privately and give advice without the parents present, unless the situation is imminently dangerous. Drugs and alcohol can slow down the recovery of the brain from injury. Tell this to the patient clearly and in simple language ("Vitamin S").

(3) Peer influences may have a big impact on return-to-play decision-making. Athletes may really want to go back to

play so that they can spend time with their teammates. Ask the patient to bring in one or a few teammates and educate them about concussion. *The no return to play within 24 hours rule, however, should be followed strictly*; adolescents with a second impact within 24 hours of concussion have a delayed recovery (Terwilliger et al., Journal of Neurotrauma, 2016). The devastating (though fortunately rare) second impact syndrome has been reported mainly in adolescents.

(4) Drug dosing for full-grown adolescents can be similar to adults, but lower doses may be required for smaller adolescents. If in doubt, consult a pediatrician or pharmacist for specific drug dosing.

(5) The late effects of complex concussion or multiple concussions in adolescence on the future development of cognitive function and emotional regulation are not well known. Therefore, consider offering long-term follow-up (1, 2, 3 years after concussion) just in case issues arise later. Even if it is not clear whether the late issues are directly caused by the concussion, they still may be treatable.

(6) Preexisting attention deficit and learning disabilities can get substantially worse after concussion. This may require intensification of pharmacological therapy (e.g., increase in stimulant dose), coordination with school special education programs, and consultation with other treating physicians.

(7) It can be hard to tell whether mood instability and conflict with parents should be attributed to concussion or to "normal teenage behavior." It doesn't really matter. If these problems are substantially impairing the patient's function or the family dynamics, treat them the same way regardless of the cause, and tell the parents "it's usually some of both." Most of the treatments are nonpharmacological, and mood stabilizing antiepileptic medications such as lamotrigine (Lamictal) and oxcarbazepine (Trileptal) have a well-established safety record in adolescents.

(8) Education of patients, parents, and peers about bicycle helmet safety, seatbelts, and the risks of teenage "fooling

around" is important to prevent recurrent concussion. Consider an empathetic approach with the adolescent. ("It's not fair, and I wish it weren't this way, but you may not be able to get away with the same kind of fooling around as your friends because you've had this concussion.") There is also emerging evidence that problem-solving training for adolescents can be helpful. Whether the parents should or should not be involved seems to depend on the level of stress within the relationships (Wade et al., Journal of Developmental & Behavioral Pediatrics, 2018).

(9) For the concussed 15- to 16-year-old patient on the cusp of starting to drive, consider advising extra caution. Go back to the beginning of driver's education and get a professional driving evaluation (see Chapter 28) with the parent riding along before taking the official driving test. Driving can be impaired even when the patient is completely asymptomatic.

(10) Adolescents may not be able to formulate questions as clearly as adults. Consider preemptively addressing questions that the adolescent may be afraid to ask. Questions such as these:

"What happens if I am still having really bad headaches, I don't tell anyone, and I get another concussion?" (*Answer: Your recovery may be a lot slower after a second concussion, and there is a risk of second impact syndrome, which can be fatal*).

"Will I be stupid for the rest of my life?" (*Answer: not likely. Most people make a very good cognitive recovery.*)

"I'm really anxious, and pot is the only thing that helps. Is that OK?"(*Answer: we have a lot more effective treatments for anxiety than pot.*)

(11) Possible role for glucose (e.g., 100 to 200 calories of a high-glycemic-index snack or drink) to improve cognitive performance. This seems to be specific to children, but it is not clear whether it benefits adolescents. May not be effective in adults.

(12) Concussion in adolescence is associated with modestly increased likelihood of developing multiple sclerosis, especially after more than 1 concussion (Montgomery et al., Annals of Neurology, 2017). The order of causality is not yet clear, but it is possible that autoimmune processes could be set into motion by concussion. On one hand, the future risk of multiple sclerosis could provide further motivation to reduce risky behavior. On the other hand, this future risk could trigger excessive anxiety. Some judgment is required to determine what to tell an adolescent patient.

35

Concussion in Children

The advice of Dr. Mark Halstead at Washington University, Dr. Chris Giza at the University of California, Los Angeles, and Dr. Gerry Gioia at Children's National Hospital regarding this section is gratefully acknowledged.

Many aspects of concussion management in children under 12 years of age are similar to the management of older patients, but there are several *special rules*:

(1) Take the history twice: Once from the child and once from the parents or guardians.

(2) Assess the maturity of the child. Young kids can reliably report only a few symptoms. All the rest of the concerns should be assessed by asking the parents or guardians. The most reliable symptoms are:
   a. Headache
   b. Nausea
   c. Balance problems
   d. Problems concentrating
   e. Irritability

(3) Use age-appropriate language with the child, as well as simplified assessments of severity.
   a. "Does your head hurt?" "Does it hurt a little or a lot?" (see Figure 35.1)
   b. "Do you feel like you are going to throw up, going to get sick?"
   c. "Are you having problems walking straight? Are you falling down more?"

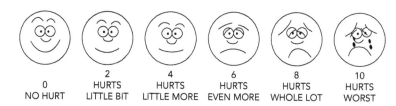

FIGURE 35.1 Wong-Baer Pain FACES Pain Rating Scale.

From Wong D. L., Hockenberry-Eaton M., Wilson D., Winkelstein M.L., Schwartz P.: *Wong's Essentials of Pediatric Nursing, Sixth Edition*, St. Louis, 2001, p. 1301. Copyrighted by Mosby, Inc. Reprinted by permission.

      d. "Are you having problems paying attention to things? Do you 'space out' more than before?"
      e. "Are you grumpy or grouchy? Having problems getting along with people?"

Consider using the Child SCAT5 (Davis et al., British Journal of Sports Medicine, 2017) for relatively acute concussions in children age 5 to 12 years.
    https://bjsm.bmj.com/content/bjsports/early/2017/04/26/bjsports-2017-097492childscat5.full.pdf
For later stages, a more individualized approach may be needed.

  (4) Get a careful history from the parents or guardians about preinjury characteristics, especially attention deficit, learning disabilities, anxiety, headaches, and seizures.
  (5) Carefully assess for secondary-gain factors. A child may either over- or under-report symptoms to please the parents or guardians. Getting a lot of extra attention from adults can be a big secondary gain in itself.
  (6) With regard to return to school, sports, and daily life, help the parents or guardians find the "middle way": Not too protective and not too lax (also known as "baby bears porridge: not too hot and not too cold . . . just right."). Consider

using the Acute Concussion Evaluation (ACE) Care Plan developed at Children's National Medical Center and the University of Pittsburgh. https://www.cdc.gov/headsup/pdfs/providers/ace_care_plan_school_version_a.pdf

a. Excessively nervous parents and guardians need to be reassured.

    i. Most children will make a good recovery.

    ii. Most symptoms will recede or become manageable.

    iii. It's OK to check on the child's symptoms once a day, checking every hour doesn't help.

    iv. Most children do not need to be "cocooned" or totally isolated from all stimuli. The main exception is when headaches are so severe that the child cannot tolerate any noise, sound, or cognitive activity. A recent randomized controlled trial of 2 days rest versus 5 days rest after concussion revealed better outcomes with 2 days rest (Thomas et al., Pediatrics, 2015).

b. Excessively unconcerned parents and guardians need to take concussion seriously, so that they don't allow their child to do something dangerous.

    i. Sometimes the term "concussive traumatic brain injury" can be used to give the event a sense of perspective.

    ii. A small amount of "Vitamin S" (the therapeutic scare), with the child out of the room, describing the second impact syndrome can be helpful for parents or guardians who push their kids to return to contact sports right away.

c. Every parent or guardian needs to be educated with regard to concussion prevention.

    i. Car safety: seat belts, car seats, no driving when distracted, keep tires well-maintained, airbags, traction control, antilock brakes, etc.

    ii. Bicycle helmets

    iii. Helmets for other sports, such as skiing, skateboarding, or horseback riding.

    iv. Watch the child more carefully until he or she has fully recovered. The child's balance and judgment may be impaired, which leads to a high risk of repeat concussion during potentially dangerous activities, such as tree climbing, rough play, or skateboard tricks.

  d. In-home family training provided by a therapist can improve outcomes for children with prolonged effects of brain injuries. Family training may be especially helpful in unstable family situations or those characterized by excessively lax or excessively rigid parenting style.

(7) *Atypical presentations of migraine.* Ask about intermittent nausea, stomach pain, or vomiting even without headache. Treat with low-dose amitriptyline at bedtime plus ibuprofen or acetaminophen as soon as possible on onset of symptoms. A great deal of experience indicates that these are safe and effective in children. Most doses of medication are based on weight: consult with a pediatrician for exact dosing.

(8) *Atypical presentations of depression and anxiety.* Ask about interpersonal problems with friends, temper tantrums, and regression of milestones. Refer to a pediatric psychologist and possibly also a pediatric psychiatrist: behavioral interventions are first-line therapy. Less is known about the effects of pharmacological treatments for depression and anxiety in children compared to adults.

(9) *Attention deficit.* Children with preinjury attention deficit, even if it was not formally diagnosed or being actively treated, can have a worsening of attention after concussion.

(10) *Executive function problems.* These can include issues with organization and planning, working memory, initiation, monitoring one's own progress, impulse control, transitioning from one activity to the next, responding appropriately, anticipating future events, and keeping track of

the effects of one's own behavior on others. Problems with executive function can be a big impediment to successful return to school. They are not always obvious right away. Take a careful history from parents and teachers. Consider using a quantitative measure such as the Behavior Rating Inventory of Executive Function (BRIEF), which is a very well validated set of questions for parents and teachers that takes about 10 to 15 minutes to administer on paper or on-line. There is a small charge for the test. https://www.parinc.com/Products/Pkey/23

(11) Possible role for *glucose* (e.g., 100 to 200 calories of a high glycemic index snack or drink 20 minutes prior to school or rehabilitation-related activity) to improve cognitive performance and reduce pain. This seems to be specific to children and does not appear to be effective in adults.

(12) *"Spells"*: After concussion, some children have short periods of unresponsiveness or interruption in their ongoing activities.

    a. First, take the history from someone who has actually seen the event, often a teacher or a friend. Have the differential diagnosis in mind while you take the history and ask specific questions:

        i. *Fainting or vasovagal syncope.* A feeling of light-headedness, vision going gray or dark, sometimes nausea, then loss of consciousness, which recovers quickly with no residual problems once the patient lies down. This is usually not a sign of a serious underlying condition. It is mainly due to dehydration, fear, or pain. Rarely, there is an underlying cardiac arrhythmia. Check a 12-lead electrocardiogram (ECG) on everyone and order a cardiac Holter-type monitor for anyone with a personal or family history of cardiac arrhythmia.

        ii. *Attention lapse.* The patient "spaces out," that is, loses his or her train of thought and briefly may be unresponsive with no memory of what was said or what happened. But then the patient has no residual problems. Attention deficit is common in children and often undiagnosed. The child may have had symptoms of attention deficit with or without hyperactivity prior to the concussion, but the symptoms can be made worse by the injury. Refer to a qualified pediatrician who treats attention deficit. Typically, this involves nonpharmacological approaches (physical exercise, attention training), pharmacological treatments (stimulants, etc.), and school accommodations. Note that a diet low in refined sugar has *not* been shown to improve attention deficit, and in fact, glucose may temporarily improve cognitive performance in children (see earlier comments).

iii. *New-onset events concerning for seizures.* Red flags:
   1. The child is truly unresponsive for more than a few seconds (not just "spacing out").
   2. The child falls badly (not a gentle collapse as in fainting).
   3. The child has eyelid movements, eye deviation to one side, facial twitching, or other repetitive movements during the spell.

Order a baseline 20-minute electroencephalogram (EEG). The EEG won't usually catch one of the spells, but if there is an abnormal background rhythm this could indicate an underlying predisposition to seizure disorder, which was likely present before the concussion but unmasked by the injury. In this case, refer to a pediatric neurologist.

If the spells are very frequent, such as several times per day, and are interfering with activities, then admit the child to the hospital for video EEG monitoring. This is the only sure way to determine whether these spells are epileptic in origin.

A worsening of preinjury seizures, absence or complex partial. Some kids with preinjury seizure disorders will have an increase in seizure frequency after a concussion. Often a small increase in the dose of usual medication for 1 to 2 weeks will be sufficient to address this. The child will likely need extra rest and may be somewhat sedated by the increased dose in medication.

36

Special Topics in Contact Sport Athletes and Others Who Have Had Multiple Concussions and Subconcussive Impacts

This area has received a lot of attention in the media, but there isn't much science.

(1) *When to retire from contact sports?* Help the patient, family, and peers think through the decision carefully. Educate them about the risk of serious and currently untreatable long-term problems, such as Chronic Traumatic Encephalopathy. Ask the following questions:

    a. "Are you going to become a professional athlete? If not, think hard about whether this is worth it." Sometimes it is. Sometimes the patient loves the sport so much that it is worth the risk.

    b. "Do you have other interests or career goals that require good cognitive abilities and interpersonal skills?" Patients usually already understand the risk of losing cognitive function, but they are less frequently aware of the risk of losing interpersonal skills, or developing depression and mood instability.

    c. "Are you interested in having a family, and maintaining good personal relations with them?" Again, many young patients haven't really thought through the effects that repeated concussions may have on their future ability to maintain good personal relationships.

As discussed in Chapter 30, after a complex concussion from which the patient is not making a rapid and complete recovery, consider strongly advising combative sport athletes such as professional boxers and mixed martial arts fighters to retire. The risk of further concussions is very high, and the potential long-term adverse effects are well-documented. In these cases, consider administering a big dose of "Vitamin S" (the therapeutic scare) by telling the patient and collateral source about the *possible* long-term effects of multiple concussions, such as chronic traumatic encephalopathy.

(2) *Does the patient have Chronic Traumatic Encephalopathy (CTE)?* There is no way to tell for sure while the patient is alive. No fixed number of concussions or subconcussive impacts are required, and there is no age cutoff. But certain features raise concerns. Obtain a focused history from a reliable collateral source and get a good quality (noncontrast) magnetic resonance imaging (MRI) scan of the brain.

Higher Concern for Chronic Traumatic Encephalopathy	*Lower Concern for Chronic Traumatic Encephalopathy*
Progressively worsening function over years to decades (but also look for other causes such as sleep deprivation, drugs and alcohol, medications)	Stable or improving function over time. (It is not known whether waxing and waning function is part of the presentation of CTE)
Mood instability, social isolation, depression, poor decision-making, and bizarre behavior are prominent.	Memory loss prominent in a very old patient is more likely to be Alzheimer's disease; refer to a memory and aging clinic. However, CTE has been reported to present as memory loss in people in their fifties through seventies.

Higher Concern for Chronic Traumatic Encephalopathy	Lower Concern for Chronic Traumatic Encephalopathy
Parkinson's-like signs: tremor, slow movements, increased resistance to passive range-of-motion testing, shuffling walk, slurred speech, reduced facial expressions, reduced blink rate, and so forth. (Also look for other causes, however, such as neuroleptics or antinausea medications)	Stiffness and slowness of movements due to musculoskeletal injuries.
Cavum septum pellucidum on MRI scan. Best seen on a high spatial resolution T1 weighted scan. Not always present, but quite common. Atrophy is only a feature of late CTE. Absence of either cavum septum pellucidum or atrophy does not rule out CTE.	Large ventricles out of proportion to sulci present on MRI or CT scan. This suggests normal pressure hydrocephalus as a possible explanation for cognitive decline and Parkinsonian features. Refer to a neurologist or neurosurgeon with expertise in normal pressure hydrocephalus.

If there is concern for CTE, treat the symptoms and do everything possible to improve quality of life. Encourage the patient to consider participating in research studies. Do not give any definite diagnosis or prognosis, given that it isn't possible to do so accurately yet. There are no specific treatments.

37

Concussion in Military Personnel

Both civilian and military doctors are increasingly seeing military patients with long-term effects of concussions. Here, the best collateral source may be another service member with whom the patient has served. Some military personnel are not fully open with their families and nonmilitary friends.

(1) Evaluate for post-traumatic stress disorder (PTSD) and treat it aggressively (see Chapter 12). Concussion and PTSD very commonly co-occur. Don't worry too much about which specific symptoms are due to traumatic brain injury (TBI) and which to PTSD. It is impossible to be absolutely sure, and the treatments for the specific symptoms are very similar, regardless of the cause. However, treatment with selective serotonin reuptake inhibitors (SSRIs) that impair sexual performance such as fluoxetine (Prozac), paroxetine (Paxil), sertraline (Zoloft), citalopram (Celexa), and escitalopram (Lexapro) is often not going to go well. Many members of the military are well aware of these side effects and may tell you they are taking them, but actually are not doing so. Behavioral therapy, prazosin, low-dose antipsychotics, and emergency benzodiazepines are often used.

(2) Evaluate for depression and treat it aggressively (see Chapter 11). Depression and PTSD occur together and can substantially increase the risk of suicide. Same issue with SSRIs that impair sexual performance. Cognitive behavioral therapy, cardiovascular exercise, and venlafaxine (Effexor) are often used.

(3) Evaluate for chronic pain and treat it aggressively (see Chapter 7). Concussion, PTSD, and chronic pain are called the "triad" because they occur together so often.

(4) Maintain confidentiality. If the patient has been using drugs and/or alcohol, it may be wise to refer them for rehabilitation discretely. Think carefully before putting this information into the medical record because active duty military personnel do not have the same privacy protections that civilians have, and this can jeopardize their future careers.

(5) Resiliency training should be specifically tailored to military service members because of the special challenges of deployment, combat, and other specific threats. The military-specific *Deployment Risk and Resilience Inventory* can be used to systematically assess resilience. https://www.ptsd.va.gov/professional/assessment/deployment/index.asp

(6) Ask specifically about number of hours slept per night and caffeine use. Excessive caffeine use and chronic sleep deprivation are epidemic in the military. Many service members may think it is normal to sleep 4 to 5 hours per night and may not realize that optimal recovery from concussion often requires 8 or more hours per night. Educate the patient, family, and fellow service members.

(7) In patients with blast-related injury or repeated low-level blast exposure, evaluate hearing carefully (see Chapter 22). Blast-related injury to the middle and inner ear is common and blast injuries affect hearing more commonly than other types of head trauma.

(8) In patients with blast-related injury or repeated low-level blast exposure, assess for tinnitus (see Chapter 22). Tinnitus is common, and effective treatment can improve quality of life.

(9) In patients with blast-related injury, evaluate balance carefully. Blast-related injury to the cerebellum is also common, and impaired balance may be more common and more severe than in other types of head trauma.

(10) Return to duty is very tricky in some cases, because of the inherent danger to the patient and to others. Return-to-duty decision-making is best done in collaboration with military physicians and occupational therapists. Civilian physicians and occupational therapists may not have the expertise or security clearance to actually understand the nature of the work, but military providers may not have the specific expertise in complex concussion management. Good communication is key. It's OK to make the patient wait while you get the right person on the phone to help sort it out.

(11) Consider treating acute blast-related concussion patients with N-acetyl cysteine (NAC) when starting within 72 hours after injury. An oral loading dose of 4000 mg followed by 2000 mg twice daily for 4 days, then 1500 mg twice daily for 3 days was shown to reduce symptom burden and to speed recovery (Hoffer et al., PLoS One, 2013). The effects of NAC on other types of concussions or at later times following injury are not known.

(12) There are many community resources specifically dedicated to wounded warriors. Become aware of what is available locally and refer the most challenging cases to the National Intrepid Center of Excellence (NICoE) in Bethesda, Maryland or to one of the Intrepid Spirit Centers on bases around the United States (See Section IV, Internet Resources). Currently, there are Intrepid Spirit Centers in Fort Belvoir, Virginia; Camp Lejeune, North Carolina; Fort Campbell, Kentucky; Fort Bragg, North Carolina; Fort Hood, Texas; Joint Base Lewis–McChord, Washington; and Camp Pendleton, California. https://www.fallenheroesfund.org/intrepid-spirit

PART III

HOW TO SET UP AND RUN A CONCUSSION CLINIC

38

Staffing

A good concussion clinic needs additional staff besides the treating providers.

First rule: Pick the right people. A concussion clinic is not for everyone. It requires greater than average interpersonal skills to handle patients with mood instability and cognitive impairment. In practical terms, this means that the people you pick need to be able to take getting yelled at by irritable patients, tolerate being cried to by depressed patients, patiently resend prescriptions and paperwork for patients who have lost them, and calmly explain things several times to worried family members. When you interview staff candidates, make it clear up front what they should expect. It helps (but is not required) to have clinic staff members who personally know someone with a history of concussion or another related neurological condition.

The clinic will need to fill the following roles:

(1) Clinic administrator to handle referrals, scheduling, phone calls, faxes, e-mails, billing, paperwork, medical records, etc. *The clinic administrator needs to have good judgment.* The administrator needs to be able to determine whether to contact the provider right away for an urgent issue, whether to recommend that the patient go straight to an emergency department, or whether a patient would be more appropriate for another clinic (e.g., orthopedic, psychiatric, neurosurgical). For a busy clinic, the clinic administrator may also need an assistant.

(2) Receptionist to check patients in, hand out self-report symptom questionnaires and other paper work, and then set up follow-up appointments, testing, etc.

(3) Nurse or nurse's aide to take vital signs, go over questionnaires, and obtain medication lists. The nurse or nurse's aide can start putting this information into the electronic medical record.

(4) Option: An in-clinic physical therapist to perform balance testing and exertional testing. A good physical therapist can also provide basic education regarding pain control, help develop an appropriate cardiovascular exercise program, and help arrange the right referrals to treating therapists. Physical therapists can bill separately from the main clinic provider.

(5) Option: An in-clinic psychometrician to perform brief cognitive testing, either traditional or computer-based. Psychometrician services can be billed separately.

(6) Option: Case manager or social worker. Often the case manager or social worker will sit in on the visit with the provider to understand the plan. He or she will expedite testing, referrals, prescriptions, and orders. He or she can help educate the patient and collateral sources further and can answer questions that didn't get asked during the visit. The case manager or social worker can be another point of contact for follow-up to make sure the plan is going well.

(7) Option: Transcriptionist to handle dictated medical records. Teach the transcriptionist the specific vocabulary used in a concussion clinic and the specific format the clinic prefers for medical records. This saves a tremendous amount of time compared with the provider typing notes or the clinic using a general transcription service without specific knowledge about concussion clinic.

(8) Option: Public relations manager to disseminate information about the clinic to potential patients and referring providers. People often hear about a concussion clinic from other patients in a support group, from a website, or from another organization. A clinic website can provide information to patients and referring providers as well as links to other resources.

(9) Option: Research coordinator. There is a boom in concussion research, and a dedicated research coordinator can help match patients with appropriate open protocols. Patients often like participating in research studies because they get more attention and may receive a new therapy. Many patients feel a sense of satisfaction at doing something for others. They get it when you tell them, "this is not about you, it's about all the other people in the future."

Second rule: Train the staff properly right from the beginning.

(1) The staff should read this manual, too, to get an idea of what sort of issues the patients and families will be concerned about.

(2) The staff should have access to other resources that the providers consider appropriate: websites, support groups, books written for the general public, other providers available for a second opinion, and so forth.

(3) The providers and staff should spend some time going over the flow of the clinic and answering questions about likely types of challenging patients—irritable, depressed, in pain, forgetful, and so on.

(4) The staff should have a clear understanding of the importance of collateral source information. In practical terms, this means making sure that the person identified as the collateral source comes to the appointment. For example, the clinic administrator or assistant may have to make two reminder phone calls: one to the patient and one to the collateral source.

(5) The providers should educate the staff to preemptively dispel some of the myths about concussion. Even well-meaning staff members may have ideas about concussion based on commonly held beliefs that are not accurate.

(6) The providers should set a clear and consistent policy with regard to prescription refills, especially for controlled

substances such as stimulants. This takes the burden off of the staff members with regard to demanding patients.

Third rule: Keep the staff happy so that you don't have high turnover. Patients and family members will get to know the staff of the clinic and come to trust and rely on them, so continuity of care with regard to the staff is important. They will be asked to do more and take on harder problems than in most clinics, so they should be appropriately compensated and treated well. Be understanding. Everyone makes mistakes and there is no "right answer" a lot of the time.

39

Typical Flow for a Concussion Clinic

Successful concussion clinics can run many different ways. In the St. Louis clinic, an initial office visit usually goes like this:

(1) Patient is referred to the clinic. The initial referral is handled by the clinic administrator. Some patients are referred by another provider, some are self-referred. Some appointments are made by a family member or collateral source, rather than by the patient. Some referrals come by phone, some by fax, some by e-mail. The administrator should be prepared for all of these.

Important: The clinic administrator needs to have good judgment. If the referral clearly indicates an urgent neurosurgical, psychiatric, or orthopedic issue, the clinic administrator should quickly make that clear to the referring provider, patient, or other referral source. The clinic administrator should have an open line of communication to the provider to help with these decisions. Text messaging (without protected health information) works especially well.

(2) Clinic administrator contacts the referring provider, patient, or collateral source and requests medical records, if not already available.

(3) Provider reviews the records and approves initial office visit if the records indicate that the patient may have had a concussion and there isn't another clinic or provider that would

be obviously more appropriate (e.g., neurosurgery, psychiatry, orthopedic surgery).

(4) Clinic administrator schedules the initial office visit. There should be two types of initial office visits at the clinic: routine and semiurgent.

    a. A routine initial office visit may involve chronic concussion-related concerns that have been relatively stable and no specific time-sensitive issues.

    b. A semiurgent initial office visit (usually within a few days of referral) may involve more recent concussion-related concerns that are not resolving as expected, symptoms that are worsening or causing substantial distress, or a time-sensitive issue such as return to work, return to school, return to duty, or return to play.

(5) Clinic administrator makes sure that the patient brings a reliable collateral source. Ideally, this is someone who knew the patient well before the injury and has a clear understanding of how the patient is doing afterward.

(6) Clinic administrator sends written date, time, and place information about the appointment to the patient *and to the collateral source*.

(7) Clinic administrator reminds the patient *and the collateral source* the day before the appointment.

(8) Patient checks in. Receptionist distributes *Rivermead Post-Concussive Symptoms Questionnaire* (http://www.tbi-impact. org/cde/mod_templates/12_F_06_Rivermead.pdf

The *Neurobehavioral Symptom Inventory (NSI)* is also commonly used http://dvbic.dcoe.mil/files/DVBIC_-_NSI_Information_Paper_Final.pdf

(9) Nurse takes temperature, blood pressure, heart rate, oxygen saturation, respiratory rate, height, and weight.

(10) Nurse collects medication list and inquires about allergies to medications.

(11) Provider obtains history and exam. Initial documentation is recorded on a preprinted sheet outlining the most important issues following concussion.

(12) Physical therapist and psychometrician see the patient. (Provider sees 1 to 2 follow-up patients in the meantime.)

(13) Provider reviews the data from the physical therapist and psychometrician.

(14) Provider performs additional testing and obtains additional history, formulates assessment, and discusses plans with patient and collateral source.

(15) Provider gives the patient and collateral source a brief handwritten or printed summary of the assessment and plan.

(16) Receptionist schedules ancillary testing and follow-up.

(17) Provider dictates notes; typically same day as clinic.

(18) Transcriptionist transcribes notes; typically 1 to 3 days after dictation

(19) Provider edits notes; typically 1 week after office visit.

(20) Transcriptionist sends notes to referring providers and others (patients themselves, lawyers, insurance companies, workman's compensation, or school administrators) as appropriate.

(21) Clinic administrator forwards e-mails, phone calls, test results, and so forth to provider by e-mail or electronic medical record tasking system.

(22) Clinic administrator sends monthly prescriptions for controlled substances if necessary.

The Walter Reed National Military Medical Center traumatic brain injury (TBI) clinic has expert case managers and social workers who coordinate care across multiple providers. This is a great benefit to patients who have often traveled a great distance for the appointment. Often, several issues are addressed in the same visit, as opposed to focusing on 1 thing at a time, and it gets pretty complicated.

40

Scheduling Return Visits

Active, immediately dangerous issue: (example: acutely suicidal or homicidal, insists on driving and clearly not able to do so safely with no way to effectively take away driving privileges.)	*Admit to hospital*
Active, time-sensitive issue: (example: professional athlete or military service member, currently unable to return to duty)	*Within 1 week*
Active, potentially dangerous issue: (example: major depression or severe anxiety, not currently suicidal)	*1 to 3 weeks*
Active, severely impairing issue: (example: severe migraine, starting on prophylactic and abortive therapy)	*1 to 2 months.*
Patient starting a new medication that requires monitoring. Examples:	*1 week to 3 months*
Starting stimulants in a patient with a history of hypertension	1 week
Starting amitriptyline (Elavil) for migraine prophylaxis	6 weeks
Starting lamotrigine (Lamictal) in a patient with nondangerous mood instability	3 months
Typical patient with moderate issues: (example: patient with cognitive impairment starting occupational therapy to assist with return to work)	*3 months*

Stable patient, medications requiring monitoring: (example: patient on stable dose of stimulants for attention deficit)	*6 months*
Stable patient, no new medications, and no medication requiring monitoring:	*1 year*

ADDITIONAL RESOURCES

Internet-based Resources

- American Academy of Neurology http://www.aan.com/concussion
- Brain Injury Association of America http://www.biausa.org/
- Brain Trauma Foundation www.braintrauma.org/
- Buffalo Concussion Treadmill Test http://www.biact.org/assets/uploads/files/Conference/Annual%20Conference%20Archives/Buffalo%20Concussion%20Treadmill%20Test%20Manual%20-%20edits.pdf
- Centers for Disease Control https://www.cdc.gov/headsup/index.html
- Defense Centers of Excellence for Psychological Health and Traumatic Brain Injury Case Management of Concussion/Mild TBI Guidance Document http://dvbic.dcoe.mil/files/TBI_CM-SOP-2013revisions-V0-6_6-5-2013.pdf
- Defense and Veterans Brain Injury Center http://www.dvbic.org/
- Intrepid Spirit Centers https://www.fallenheroesfund.org/intrepid-spirit
- National Football League Concussion Policy: http://www.nflevolution.com/
- National Intrepid Center of Excellence: http://www.wrnmmc.capmed.mil/NICoE/SitePages/index.aspx

- Rocky Mountain Hospital for Children Concussion Management Program http://www.rockymountainhospitalforchildren.com/sports-medicine/concussion-management/reap-guidelines.htm
- Veterans Administration https://www.healthquality.va.gov/guidelines/Rehab/mtbi/
- University of Pittsburgh Sports Medicine Concussion Program http://rethinkconcussions.upmc.com/
- Zurich consensus statement on concussion in sport: http://bjsm.bmj.com/content/47/5/250.full

Concussion-related Scales and Scores

Acute Concussion Evaluation (ACE)
https://www.cdc.gov/headsup/pdfs/providers/ace-a.pdf
Balance Error Scoring System (BESS)
http://fs.ncaa.org/Docs/health_safety/BESS%20manual%20
    310.pdf
Behavior Rating Inventory of Executive Function (BRIEF)
https://www.parinc.com/Products/Pkey/24
Child Sports Concussion Assessment Tool–5th Edition
    (Child SCAT5)
https://bjsm.bmj.com/content/bjsports/early/2017/04/26/
    bjsports-2017-097492childscat5.full.pdf
Deployment Risk and Resilience Inventory https://www.ptsd.
    va.gov/professional/assessment/deployment/index.asp
Epworth Sleepiness Scale
http://yoursleep.aasmnet.org/pdf/Epworth.pdf
Fatigue Severity Scale
http://geriatrictoolkit.missouri.edu/fatigue/Fatigue-Severity-
    Scale.pdf
Headache Impact Test (HIT6)
http://neurohealth.info/wp-content/uploads/2010/10/hit6.pdf
Insomnia Severity Index

https://www.myhealth.va.gov/mhv-portal-web/insomnia-severity-index

Migraine Disability Assessment Test (MIDAS)
https://migraine.com/wp-content/uploads/2012/04/midas.pdf

Military Acute Concussion Evaluation (MACE)
https://prolongedfieldcare.files.wordpress.com/2014/11/mace.pdf

Montreal Cognitive Assessment (MoCA)
http://www.memorylosstest.com/dl/moca-test-english-7-1.pdf

Neurobehavioral Symptom Inventory (NSI)
http://dvbic.dcoe.mil/files/DVBIC_-_NSI_Information_Paper_Final.pdf

Patient Health Questionnaire 9 (PHQ9) for Depression
https://www.uptodate.com/contents/calculator-depression-screening-by-a-nine-item-patient-health-questionnaire-phq-9-in-adults

http://www.cqaimh.org/pdf/tool_phq9.pdf

PTSD Checklist for DSM-5 (PCL-5)
https://www.ptsd.va.gov/professional/assessment/adult-sr/ptsd-checklist.asp

Rivermead Post-Concussion Symptoms Questionnaire
http://www.tbi-impact.org/cde/mod_templates/12_F_06_Rivermead.pdf

Sport Concussion Assessment Tool 5th Edition (SCAT5)
https://bjsm.bmj.com/content/bjsports/early/2017/04/26/bjsports-2017-097506SCAT5.full.pdf

Vestibular Ocular Motor Screening (VOMS)
http://rethinkconcussions.upmc.com/2016/10/what-is-voms/
https://www.physiotherapyalberta.ca/files/vomstool.pdf

Wong-Baker Pain Faces for Kids
http://www.wongbakerfaces.org/

Additional Publications for More Detailed Information

- *Concussion: A Clinical Profile Approach to Assessment and Treatment,* A. Kontos & M. Collins, American Psychological Association, 2018
- *Sports Concussions: A Complete Guide to Recovery and Management,* I. Gagnon & A. Ptito, CRC Press, 2017
- *Sports-Related Concussion: Diagnosis and Management,* 2nd Edition, B. Sindelar & J.E. Bailes, CRC Press, 2017
- *Brain Injury Medicine: Principles and Practice,* 2nd Edition, N. Zasler, D. Katz, R. Zafonte, D. Arciniegas, M. Bullock, & J. Kreutzer, Demos Medical Publishing, 2012
- *Handbook of Headache,* 2nd Edition, R.W. Evans & N.T. Mathew, Lippincott Williams & Wilkins, 2004
- *Localization in Clinical Neurology,* 7th Edition, P.W. Brazis, J.C. Masdeu, & J. Biller, Lippincott Williams & Wilkins, 2016 (contains especially detailed section on cranial nerve injury)
- *Manual of Traumatic Brain Injury Management,* F.S. Zollman, Demos Medical Publishing, 2011
- *Mild Traumatic Brain Injury and Postconcussion Syndrome: The New Evidence Base for Diagnosis and Treatment,* M.A. McCrea, Oxford University Press, 2007

- *Pediatric and Adolescent Concussion: Diagnosis, Management, and Outcomes*, J.N. Apps & K.D. Walter, Springer, 2012
- *Textbook of Traumatic Brain Injury*, 2nd Edition, edited by J.M. Silver, T.W. McAllister, & S.C. Yudofsky, American Psychiatric Publishing, 2011
- *Wolff's Headache and Other Head Pain*, 8th Edition, S.D. Silberstein, R.B. Lipton, & D.W. Dodick, Oxford University Press, 2007

Suggested Reading for Patients and Families

- *Getting Better (and Better) after Brain Injury: The Survivor's Guide for Living Smarter and Happier*, 2nd Edition, J. Kreutzer, E. Godwin, K. Wilder-Schaaf, & M. Wetsel, The National Resource Center for Traumatic Brain Injury, 2012
- The University of Pittsburgh Sports Medicine Concussion Program http://rethinkconcussions.upmc.com/
Rocky Mountain Hospital for Children Concussion Management Program
- http://www.rockymountainhospitalforchildren.com/sports-medicine/concussion-management/ParentRecommendations 10%2013.pdf

Suggestions, corrections, comments, and questions for the author david.brody@usuhs.edu

Glossary of Terms and Abbreviations

ACE	Acute Concussion Evaluation
BESS	Balance Error Scoring System
BRIEF	Behavior Rating Inventory of Executive Function
Cauda equina	bundle of nerves leaving the spinal cord to innervate the lower part of the body
Cavum septum pellucidum	division of the 2 leaves of the thin membrane dividing the anterior ventricles
Cerebral edema	swelling of the brain
Concussion	a traumatic brain injury at the least dangerous end of the spectrum of severity
Contusion	bruising of the brain with a mixture of bleeding and swelling
Cribriform plate	thin bones between the nasal passages and the brain
CSF	Cerebrospinal fluid
CT	computed tomography
CTE	Chronic Traumatic Encephalopathy
ENT	an ear, nose, and throat doctor; otorhinolaryngologist
Epidural hematoma	bleeding on the outside of the dura underneath the skull

GCS	Glasgow Coma Scale: Score ranging from 3 (worst) to 15 (best) indicating the severity of an acute TBI
HIT6	Headache Impact Test
Hydrocephalus	excessive fluid in the ventricles of the brain
Intracerebral hemorrhage	bleeding inside the brain
MIDAS	Migraine Disability Assessment Test
MoCA	Montreal Cognitive Assessment
MRA	magnetic resonance angiogram
MRI	magnetic resonance imaging
NSAIDS	nonsteroidal anti-inflammatory agents
PTSD	Post-traumatic stress disorder
SCAT5	Sport Concussion Assessment Tool 5th Edition
SSRI	serotonin specific reuptake inhibitor
Subdural hematoma	bleeding on the outside of the brain underneath the dura
TBI	traumatic brain injury
Thecal sac	leathery covering of the spinal cord and cauda equina
TIA	transient ischemic attack
VOMS	Vestibular Ocular Motor Screening

Index

Tables and figures are indicated by an italic *t* and *f* following the page number.